Just ONE Thing:

Simplifying the Mystery of a Healthy Lifestyle

Just One Thing.

Copyright © 2017 by Keri Lappi

Cover design: Amie Olson
Interior design: Keri Lappi

All rights reserved. No part of this book may be reproduced in any form or by any electronic or mechanical means, including information storage and retrieval systems, without permission in writing from the author. For information, email energeticwellnesscoaching@gmail.com.

The content of this book is for general instruction only. Each person's physical, emotional, and spiritual condition is unique. The instruction in this book is not intended to replace or interrupt the reader's relationship with a physician or other professional. Please consult your doctor for matters pertaining to your specific health and diet. The intent of the author is only to offer information of a general nature to help you in your quest of well-being. In the event you use any of the information in this book for yourself, the author and the publisher assume no responsibility for your actions.

All rights reserved. No part of this publication may be reproduced, distributed, or transmitted in any form or by any means, including photocopying, recording, or other electronic or mechanical methods, without the prior written permission of the publisher or author, except in the case of brief quotations embodied in critical reviews and certain other noncommercial uses permitted by copyright law. For permission requests, email the publisher or author at energeticwellnesscoaching@gmail.com.

To contact the author, visit energeticwellnesscoaching.com

ISBN-13: 978-1543298499

ISBN-10: 1543298494

Printed in the United States of America

This book is dedicated to the many teachers I've had throughout my life.

Not all of you are teachers by profession,
but you've given to me and made my life richer:

Mr. Fred Crissey,
for calling my 8th grade English papers the Dead Sea scrolls
because I tend toward exuberantly verbose;

Dr. Vincent Lombardi,
for teaching Spartan undergraduates about life
and settling the debate about proper sock folding;

Dr. Robert Fiore,
for being the most passionate, educated, vibrant storyteller
and lover of learning and language;

Joshua Rosenthal,
for your twinkling wit and tenacity for making the world a healthier place;

my parents,
who taught me how to do everything
and always believed I could do anything; and

my husband,
who reminds me by his unwavering kindness
to be less of a jerk every single day.

CONTENTS

Help! Where do I start?   *vii*
Who are you, anyway?   *xi*

Chapter 1: Leftover Mentality   1
Chapter 2: Drink Up, Get Your Water On   10
Chapter 3: Food You Should Eat   22
Chapter 4: Quasi-Foodlike Substances That Maybe
            You Shouldn't Eat   44
Chapter 5: Probiotics   54
Chapter 6: Exercise: Pump It Up   68
Chapter 7: Stress and Self-Care   80
Chapter 8: Just Go To Sleep   90
Chapter 9: Laughter and a Positive Attitude   100
Chapter 10: Organization   114
Chapter 11: Your Kick in the Rear   124

Acknowledgements
Endnotes

Help! Where do I start?

I've heard it maybe one billion times before. The question looms over the heads of those trying to find their way through the vast myriads of whatever the heck it means to be healthy and eat in a healthy way. And to nearly everyone, it is a dark, cloudy path up the world's largest mountain. Why is it so difficult? Take one glance into the food and diet section of any bookstore, library, or website in the world and you won't wonder for more than a few seconds.

There's just so much to worry and think about.

So, where do you start? I mean, do you hit up eliminating sugar? Or do you go organic on the produce and straighten out your dirty dozen (see ewg.org for help on that)? Do you eradicate GMOs from your diet? Do you stop eating meat? Should you just remove the preservatives, or do you cut the partially hydrogenated oils, the high fructose corn syrup, the excitotoxins (MSG, aspartame), and hope for the best? What about going raw or paleo? Is it all safe to do if you have children (and they have to eat that way too?)? What about traditional or fermented foods? Or should you worry about the food later and start exercising instead? If so, what? Cardio? Weights? Both? When? How? Can't I just do a tabata class, go home, scarf a bowl of ice cream and call it even? What of all those concerns you hear about – microwave use, cell phone radiation, and whatever else out there is going to kill us.

And what of all the conflicting information? How do we reconcile that this professional is telling us that we need to eat low fat, and this researcher is saying that you should be eating more fat? How is this guy over here succeeding at the Mediterranean diet, and this one is feeling amazing on Paleo, but this one is all about raw food or Whole 30? Should I be juicing? Or is that too much sugar? Speaking of sugar, what really is sugar – am I supposed to be cutting out fruit along with my chocolate cake, or do I switch over to maple syrup or something?

Inevitably, by the time you even let your mind think through this list, you have already given up hope at the impossible dream of becoming whatever on earth it is to be healthy. Forget it all. It's just too much.

Or is it?

You do know the old saying, "Rome wasn't built in a day."

I'm here to let you know that your health and your philosophy of wellness weren't either, and it will take a little bit to squeeze out of that mindset that has been built firmly onto the metal bars of your mind.

What if you could just focus on one thing at a time? When you learned math, you weren't likely given proofs to solve and algebraic equations to decipher ahead of you learning to multiply, were you? You need logical building blocks, and once you have those, they aren't difficult anymore. They aren't something you must struggle and ponder over. They're able to become your lifestyle when you adopt them into your family slowly.

As a health coach it is my passion and my job to help people connect to a sustainable healthy lifestyle where they can make adjustments based on listening to their body's needs. I wake up every morning excited that I have the opportunity to connect people to their goals, and to the best self of who they want to be.

In my health coaching practice, I see people who have myriads of different goals – everything from weight loss, to getting off prescription meds, to having more energy, to seeking out ground level holistic solutions to their pervasive health issues, and many others. Nope, I'm not a physician, but I believe that if the body is given what it needs, it will heal itself, and I've watched it happen over and over again. We have to be able to do the hard work of silencing the voices outside and listen to what we're supposed to be doing, a practice that becomes more difficult the more plugged in our society is because everyone's needs are different. I believe in the philosophy of bio-individuality created by Joshua Rosenthal: that one person's food is another person's poison. We're all different, with different ancestry, different DNA, blood types, experiences, body images, motivations, and conditions. There are overarching principles that bring health to all humanity, but I want to teach you how to find out what your body needs and what it is saying to you.

How does this happen? That's what this book is about. When I sit down with a client, I do not have a preconceived notion about what they need, or about a plan I'm going to definitely put them on. I have to listen to them, to hear their history, the beliefs and weights that they are carrying, and to research for their needs. While I cannot know the depths of what you are going through and solve your specific issues through a book, there are universal health truths that solve a giant bulk of the issues and help people toward a sustainable and healthy lifestyle. I want to take you through the main points of what I hash out with my clients, one step at a time, to help you think about those things and to hold your hand and walk you toward who you want to be.

For the rest of the details and the next step, I highly recommend you connect with me or a certified local integrative nutrition health coach that you trust to get personal attention and accountability.

I've always wanted to save and fix the world. The information that I present to you is given with the hope that you will also be able to make sustainable change, one step at a time, so that your life can be what you've hoped it to be, and not just something akin to a Pinterest board (you know, where it looks really great, but you never get around to actually doing it?). It is my passion to educate others that they don't have to feel tired, depressed, lethargic, purposeless, sick, and sad. I envision a world where people suck the life out of life, where our lives are full of vibrancy and not just years, where people are living all of their days fulfilling their calling. Can you even imagine? I can. One day at a time, one person at a time.

I'm here to motivate and push you. Are you ready for a change? I am excited for your success. Welcome to the winning team.

Come on, let's do this.

Who are you, anyway?

I wasn't always like this. For anyone who knows me, I might be what you'd consider a Birkenstock wearing, crunchy, hemp, flax, and chia seed loving organic hippie (except in black heels, a pencil skirt, carrying a pink purse). If you knew me in high school or in college, an amused smirk would spread slowly across your face, and you would ask me if I remember one of my nicknames – Mountain Dew Girl.

Yes, it's true, the neon green, butane-filled caffeinated elixir of artificial sugars was my mojo. Let me break it down to you like this: I was on the swim team and one of the rules we had during high school season was that we had to refrain from eating blatant sugar. This was excessively distressing because Halloween falls within high school girls swimming season. Since I am a person who generally abides by the rules, I would fastidiously obey my coach throughout the season, but because of my desperate love and addiction to sugar, at the end of the season, you would find me sitting on the floor in my extra-large closet with a pillowcase full of Halloween candy, a comatose smile on my face, and an apparent war scene of 99 torn and empty wrappers littering my immediate proximity.

I went through college the same way, eating colorful sugar cereal for breakfast (and dinner, sometimes). I grew up on Twinkies, Twix, Cheese-Its, Doritos, Mountain Dew, Capri Sun, and Little Debbie cakes so I continued eating whatever I wanted without pausing for one moment to wonder what I was eating. It was on the shelf at the grocery store, so obviously it was just fine. They wouldn't sell something if they knew it was bad for you. I mean, they can't. Right?

Fast forward a few years and I'm a wife and new mom. My friend Amy tells me that she is avoiding partially hydrogenated oils and high fructose corn syrup for her husband's health. My eyebrows furrow, wait, *what?* Why is she avoiding this? She says she wants to protect his heart and the doctor said that he needed to stay away from that stuff. I had considered doing things for vanity before (like diets and exercise programs), but not for the purpose of improving my overall health. Hmm. That's a novel idea.

Am I eating this stuff? Am I giving it to my family? Shouldn't I be protecting them too? I started to research. I read up on it. I decided that if she could do it, I could do it. Kick in my competitive nature. Scratch that, I *will* do this. Project Eradicate Crappy Food was underway.

I was surprised by how many things were full of high fructose corn syrup and partially hydrogenated oils. I kept reading. Why are they allowed to sell this? If they are selling this, what else are they doing?

Thus began my gateway drug into healthy living, but more than that – I began asking questions about what is in our food, why it's there, and wondering about the link between what we consume and our health. I knew that if you eat a bunch of Taco Bell and McDonald's every day, you're going to be a fatty (with the caveat of: well, if you don't exercise, I mean), but beyond that, what was happening in our society? Everyone is so sick. I remember in elementary school someone saying that by the time we were adults, we would know someone personally who had cancer. I had scrunched up my face in disbelief and shock. Really? I think about that now and the names and faces of people I love who have heard that diagnosis and pitiably, it's more than a few. Something isn't right here.

I read and researched and got mad and passionate. People are getting sick because of what they eat and nobody is telling them. I have to tell them! I must save the world!

A few years later, I was walking in my favorite health food store and they had different people setting up small tables giving samples and talking with people. I met a woman who told me that she was a health coach. I had no idea what that was, so I asked her what she meant. She told me that she meets with people to help them to make better and healthier choices and works with them personally to educate them toward their goals and better health. My jaw dropped. That's a thing?! That was *exactly* what I wanted to do, but I thought that the way to go about that was to become a dietician or a nutritionist. I had held that lofty goal in my heart for a few years, but because I was a homeschooling stay-at-home mom, there was no way that I could get that done. The schooling wasn't reasonable, the timing wasn't good, the money wasn't there for that kind of thing.

I sped home. I ran in the house and was practically shaking with excitement over this new idea. I told my husband that this was what I wanted to do, and what someday I would do. The determined look in my eye is one that he is familiar with and he knew that even though it wasn't an option that I could pursue at that point, he knew that it was futile to try to dissuade me fully.

Years passed and I read and researched, cleaned up our food, made more and more things from scratch, spoke with others about their own health and about options that they might try through nutrition or holistic remedies. People knew that I had this passion, but it was just that. I had no formal schooling or certification. My family was healthy, my kids were smart and happy, and I finally felt like I was not hopeless and hapless in health. I had a say and I could make smart decisions. There was something comforting about realizing my fate wasn't lying in the hands of a doctor who barely had time to listen to me and saw me once a year for fifteen minutes.

There were a lot of schools that offered different things, but I wanted one with a focus on holistic health and solving problems by getting to the bottom of the issue instead of covering the symptoms of things. I found the school that I wanted to go to whenever the possibility opened into reality and I got emails from them occasionally. About three years after I met that woman and decided I was going to be a health coach, I got the news that I knew would change everything. There was a deep discount on tuition and I had to grab it. I knew that this was my chance and my time. I knew that tuition could not come out of the family budget, so I was going to have to figure it out.

I worked up a plan in my head that I would sell a bunch of Norwex and just make it happen. I would bust my rear for this dream, I didn't know how I was going to get it done, but I had to take that chance. The program counselors said that halfway through the program you could start taking clients under your provisional certificate and make some money that way to pay off your tuition. I wanted to believe it and I did. I signed up.

They were right. I completed my program through the Institute for Integrative Nutrition and by the time I graduated, I had a full health coaching practice. Through health coaching, I have been able to touch the lives of people on a personal basis and watch them grow in every way toward their goals. I've seen people go into remission from Rheumatoid Arthritis, get to their goal weight, clear their brain fog, detox excess estrogen, have more energy, get off prescription meds, pursue their career dreams, learn how to listen to their body and know what works for them, and iron out a lifestyle that is healthy, happy, and sustainable.

I want people to suck the life out of life. It's no good to merely survive. I want people to have life and health in their years, to be able to fulfill their calling, pursue their dreams with fiery passion, and serve those that they love fully. Can you imagine the world if filled with such people?

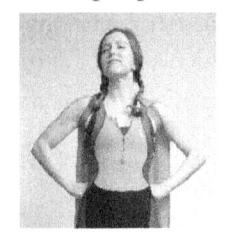

I can. And I'm determined to make it happen (in a cape if necessary).

Chapter 1: Leftover mentality

Two-week goal: To be able to plan and think ahead enough to ferociously combat "leftover mentality".

She slams the fridge shut, spins around and calls out to her children, "Hurry up! Get in the car! You're going to be late for school!" On the way out the door, she grabs a cracked piece of Pop Tart that was left on her child's plate, shoves it into her mouth, tosses the travel mug of coffee into her bag (*thank God for coffee*), and scans the room with her eyes before she locks up the door. The dishes are piled everywhere in the kitchen – the table, the counter, and the clean ones in the dishwasher need emptying. There is a pile of papers she needs to go through sitting on the desk. The clean clothes made it out in a basket, but they're lying on the couch, half folded because that's where she passed out last night watching a last few minutes of TV in an attempt to relax before bed. She furrows her brow. Everywhere she looks is a reminder of a to-do list.

As she rushes the kids into the car and makes sure they're buckled in, she pulls her seatbelt across herself and makes a face. "Ugh," she mutters to herself, "these pants don't fit anymore! I've got to do something. Maybe one of those shakes that everyone is always talking about. I'm so tired, I feel like crap, I don't like how I look in my clothes, and I'm so stressed out!" She doesn't have a lot of time to think about it, because the kids are fighting in the backseat, and she's got to go to work and deal with everything that awaits her there. She's got to push that stuff behind her and pretends she's got it together and that she's polished, because they expect her to be. She'll figure it out later. Eventually.

After work, she goes to the store and buys the usual – some cereal, frozen waffles, frozen chicken nuggets, frozen bagged dinners, some salad, juice, and some fruit. When she gets home, everyone is hungry, and she is exhausted and annoyed at the view of the chaos that is around her. She doesn't have time or energy to make dinner, so she suggests to her husband that they just grab a pizza. That sounds fine to him (because he certainly isn't going to make dinner), so they put the groceries away and try to clear up enough space to sit down at the table. She pours a glass of wine (*thank the Lord for wine*) and eats a piece of pizza. She's got to make the kid's lunches for tomorrow, and maybe arrange a yogurt and a bagel for hers, fold up the rest of the laundry, and find that permission slip for the field trip tomorrow in the pile of papers. Her husband is giving her some sassy eyebrow look and she scowls at him. (Maybe if he folded the laundry once in a while, he would have a better chance! Is he an absolute idiot not to know this?) Like she's got energy and time for that. It's going to be another long night so she can fall asleep and do it all over again in the morning.

(Insert record scratch!)

She's just living the dream, isn't she? I mean, it just sounds like absolute paradise, doesn't it?

This poor woman has no name because she could be anyone out there – male or female – rushing through life, waiting for a vacation or an extra day to catch up, hoping for a break, hoping that something will give somewhere. She doesn't exercise. She doesn't have the energy or the desire to do it, except for when she gets a quick glance at herself in the mirror on the way into the shower, and then she swears that today is the day. Well…until the specially made cookies are brought into the office and then, in that case, she'll start tomorrow.

Unfortunately, it's been "tomorrow" for a few years now and if she doesn't stop and change something, this is going to float her to the end of her life.

There are a lot of things going on here that are not working for her and serving her.

1. She's got leftover mentality.
2. She wants to make a deposit with junk and is expecting a return in gold.
3. She's not planning ahead and preparing, so life is tossing her around like a rag doll.

Let's deal with leftover mentality first. This is something I see in almost all of my mom clients, but it is prevalent in everyone. It's the mentality of making things work for everyone else and treating yourself like leftovers. It's seen in the shards of Pop Tarts that you pop into your mouth on the way out the door. It's there when you're home alone so you don't bother to make a proper lunch for yourself (since you've got no reason to, I mean, *it's just you*) so you open the fridge and eat the most random things you can find, just to make your hunger shut up. It's a yogurt and crackers for lunch because you won't have to do dishes and you can eat it fast so you can get back to the project you're in the middle of. It's not making a real dinner because your husband is gone for the evening so you can just eat some fantastically healthy thing like a box of mac and cheese and hope it will sustain your busy life for the next twelve hours.

I'm not going to go overboard and promote blatant selfishness in the me-first-me-only mentality that our world is drowning in, because I think that you have a lot to give, and I think that you should use your talents and not waste them or bottle them up. There is a narrow path that splits both sides of things: selfishness and wild gluttony on one side, and martyrdom and leftovers on the other. Neither is a healthy lifestyle and neither will give you what you need to have the energy, tenacity, and capability to achieve your goals and change the world for the better.

In exercise and physical health, this looks like you running yourself down so tired that you have no desire or ability to wake up and exercise (or carve out some time in your day to do so). It looks like you making time to go to everyone else's activities and not creating your own that pour back into your soul and body. It looks like you overbooking yourself to the point that you have to stay up very late to even feel like you're not getting too far behind in life, getting hardly any sleep, and throwing yourself into chronic tiredness (which screws up your hormones, increases your stress level, and makes it impossible for you to lose weight even when you try).

Emotionally, you hit a chain reaction because you're chronically tired and now your emotions aren't easily under your control. You're easily angered, have no patience, and push yourself to frustration, only to explode at the people closest to you, and let's not even talk about the incompetent drivers in front of you when you're already late. You feel scattered and life feels like it is spinning out of control.

It doesn't have to be like this. You can take steps to push back on the demands of life and get ahead of things. It is not rocket science, but it will take a little bit of planning. You've already proved you're capable of doing it because you do it for everyone else (see what I just did there?). You just need to listen to your body and take care of what it needs. You've got to push yourself in this area and be a good steward of the gift of your life. Other people need you. You can't treat yourself like leftovers and expect to be awesome. It won't happen.

There is no magic wand that I could wave to make you see this. You have to grab it on your own. It doesn't have to be the flip of a calendar page for you to start. It doesn't have to be a Monday. It doesn't have to be after a birthday party. It doesn't have to be because of a wedding or a cruise or a vacation in the middle of the winter. In fact, (like Mastin Kipp says) it would have been optimal for you to have started yesterday, but today will be just fine. You have to get sick enough of where you're at and tell yourself that you ought to be getting a little bit more out of life than what you are allowing. If you feel mediocre and you're happy about it, your comfort level will keep you exactly where you are. If you're walking on the beach with your friends and your thighs are chafing because you've gained weight and you can't stand it anymore, that's a great place to be. Pain will make you change.

I want you to want more than an exit strategy for your pain, though. I want you to be able to go after your goals. I want you to dream big and to decide that you're going to throw off the dead weight and do what needs to be done to step into the life that you want to live. No, you're not all-powerful, neither are you sovereign, but you do have a reasonable amount of say in the direction of where you can end up. Do you want to be happy and healthy? You can do that. It is attainable. Do you want to do the best you can to avoid illness and the diseases of your parents and grandparents? You can work at that, too. If you do nothing, you will remain as you are and float to the end of the river of your life, a passive passenger on your inner tube. Do you like this ride? Would you like to drive a little? Will you ponder it with fondness when you get to the end? If that doesn't sound like how you want to live out the rest of your life, then you need to make change. It starts with you. Get sick of where you are. Tell yourself that you're done treating yourself like crappy leftovers.

If you have to say it to yourself in the mirror every morning, do it. If you can write out a few goals every single day, do it. Speak what you intend for the day and make sure it is aligned with your weekly, monthly, yearly, and life goals. You can drive or you can be driven. Sometimes you have no choice, but when you do, I hope you are going where you need to be.

This leads into the second thing that is going on: you can't deposit junk and expect gold. Everything that you put into your body, into your life, into your workout, and into your relationships comes back to you in the way in which you deposit it. Your life is a bank. If I want to be able to run a sub seven-minute mile for a 5k, I need to work on sprints and put in the appropriate distance to be able to carry me that far. Showing up to a race and having run an average of one mile a week at a haphazard pace is not going to bring me the results I want to have, but this is exactly what a lot of people expect out of their lives, especially in the area of health. Many people expect it to be easier. It's not and that's not how it works. You can only withdraw what you've put in. Life is mostly work (unless you are a child or an adult baby). You'll be a lot happier when you wrap your arms around that fact and truly savor the moments of relaxation and enjoyment instead of expecting them. Work hard and make what you do work for you.

Let me tell you a secret, and I really want you to grasp this. It is vital to understanding why you should care about nutrition, sleep, drinking water, exercising, and the whole nine yards. Ready? You cannot produce the energy needed to do the things you want to do (and need to do) if you are haphazard in what you put into your body. If you are eating your child's leftover chicken nuggets for lunch (because they are there and check, you ate something, so you're fine for now and hey, back to folding laundry), you are not going to have enough energy to make a good and healthy dinner. When dinner time comes, you're going to want to do what is easy because you do not have the reserves to do anything else. This is a perpetual downward spiral. You don't have energy, so you eat some quick junk. Your quick junk gives you nothing nutritionally (or very little) and your body cannot properly function. You are walking into becoming chronically nutritionally deficient. Your brain cannot function well like this. You are starving it and depriving your body. You are a machine that is rusting out and your solution is to oil it up with acid rain. (How's that working out for you? What will happen to a body that keeps going like this?)

Real energy and health cannot be found in nutritionally-deficient quasi-foodlike substances. You cannot thrive when you do not have real fuel. Food is pleasurable, but food has a purpose. It is medicine to your body. It is information. It is fuel. Do not be solely ruled by the dictates of your palate (especially when your palate is not to be trusted because it's so skewed from being trained on sugar and chemicals). That is a life lacking in self-control. You can do better than that, and you deserve to choose the things that your body needs, not only the things that your taste buds want. The benefit of self-control and self-discipline are myriad, and making a better choice in this area will pay you back exponentially.

I want to help you with exactly this. Nutrition has more to do with your output than you can even begin to imagine. In the chapter on food, I'm going to give you the details about eating cleaner (and how to decipher through the seemingly conflicting information). Your energy, athletic ability, and physical health hinge upon the information you give your body through food. Every bite is a step in the direction of strength and health or a step toward disease and degeneration. This is not to say that you must always eat perfectly, but rather that you can choose to be informed so at least you can make knowledgeable decisions regarding your life and health. You know the risk in smoking cigarettes – if you choose to do it, that's up to you because you walked into that knowing exactly what to expect. In the area of food and nutrition, things are a little bit more hazy and there is a lot of marketing to make it seem that something is going to help you reach your goals, when it is only filling the deep pockets of a corporation. I want you to be able to filter through this to avoid the deception and truly feed your body.

Lastly, the red flag I see in this poor woman's day is a lack of organization and preparedness. It is difficult to always be on top of things, but it is tremendously more difficult when you have no plan or strategy for your day to do so. Life has a pile of basic requirements - you have to eat, you have to go to work (or be productive in an unpaid fashion), you have to pick up your kids, and you have to go grocery shopping – don't make it more painful for you by allowing the things that you *can control* to be completely *out of control*. You know the old cliché: if you fail to plan, you plan to fail. I want to help you with that, too. There is a chapter with specifics on organization. Check it out when you're ready.

Here is an amazing thing: when you start doing one good thing for yourself, you get a boost. Your brain and your soul start telling you that you can do things, that you've accomplished something great for yourself (even if it is a little something). Guess what happens? It's an upward spiral! You drink some water and your brain flips a switch and you're like, "Hey, I'm all healthy now! Look at me! I'm rocking this. I'm pretty much on my way to becoming an Olympic athlete, so WHAT UP NOW!" This is great. This is free inspiration and motivation and I want you to take it and fly with it. Each step you take walks you to where you want to go.

If you derail – and my darling, you will derail at times – I want you to stand right back up. Tripping is part of learning how to walk. Do you expect a toddler to be able to run as well as a Notre Dame cross country star? When we're reprogramming our behaviors, there are times that you will screw up. That is okay. Say it with me, "If I mess up, that is okay. I can restart and go in the right direction. It is not over. I did not fail because I do not fail. I win or I learn." I want you to push yourself, but I want you to realize that you're not going to be perfect (I suppose this is news to you, and I'm sorry I had to be the one to break it to you). When you make a less than optimal choice, I want you to realize it, absorb it, think about how it made you feel (and write that down so you remember), roll with it and move back onto your path. This is your path and these are your goals.

You have two little voices in your head (if you keep reading, it will be my intention to make one of those voices mine so that you will hear me standing on your shoulder when you're faced with challenging choices…muahahahaha) and the one you feed will be the one who grows and gets stronger. It is a daily choice to get up and to pursue your goals. Nobody else is going to do it for you, and the outcome of where you're going is built upon what you do today. Wake up, chin up, and push it like a hustler.

Here's how this book is going to work – every chapter starts off with a two-week goal. Read the chapter. At the end of each, there is an action step. Make the goal specific to you and your situation, and this is what you will work on for two weeks. You can stretch it out longer than that (do it for a month, etc.), but I want you to do a minimum of two weeks before you add anything else in. The goals and recommendations in the book are meant to help you toward a healthier lifestyle overall.

I want the two-week goal to become your normal. I want it to become part of your everyday not-even-thinking-about-it lifestyle. I want you to tweak it to find what works for you for the rest of your life. This is not a fad. It is absolutely useless (if not harmful) for me to push you to lose 50 pounds in a month eating cabbage soup only for you to gain 60 back, wreck your metabolism, kill your self-esteem, stress out your body, and make you do wild and unsustainable things. The recommendations in this book are not wild. They are do-able. They are sustainable. I'm not going to suggest something to you that I'm not doing or trying to do myself. You may find a certain one to be more challenging than another, but fight through this because you can win it. You're on the winning team, didn't you know?

Write down your action step where you will see it and put a reminder in your phone where you will be haunted by it daily, and then I want you to smash that goal and make it your own. Show it who is boss. It's time to set the excuses aside. They do not serve you. Let's get you where you want to be.

Ready for a pep talk? Great. Here it is: stop being a spineless wussbucket. Man up. Pull up your big girl panties and do something about it. This is your life. Make something of it and get after it.

Let's go. Your dreams and goals are waiting.

Action steps:

Read a chapter. Take action. Win at life.

The voice you feed is the one that grows stronger.

Chapter 2: Drink Up, Get Your Water On

Two Week Goal: Drink at least 16 ounces before you drink or eat anything in the morning; increase overall water consumption.

"Ugh, I literally hate water. I hate it. It's so boring. Can I put some stuff into it?" My client looked up at me, a little bugged that I told her that I was recommending that she drink 16 ounces before she did anything else in the morning. I'd heard this sentiment before – from my mother, who drinks about 4 ounces of water on a good day, but who manages to suck down two coffees before she checks out Kelly Ripa's outfit for the day.

"Just do it for these two weeks. You can do this. Come on, yank up the big girl panties and make it happen." I encouraged her. I looked across the table at my client, knowing that this was a big deal to her, but that it was also a big deal and important to get done.

If you think about it, when you wake up in the morning, it's very likely that you have not had anything to drink for a pile of hours. What do you do next? You go to the bathroom. (If you don't, you're so dehydrated that I'm dedicating this chapter to you.) Think about that. What do most people do next? They go brew a pot of coffee and start chugging. Welcome to the Usain Bolt version of running straight toward dehydration.

I have a client, Roxy*, whose 9-year-old daughter had been having headaches and stomach pains for as long as she could remember (*fake names, real peeps). She was chronically constipated, was dealing with ADD, and just felt awful most of the time. She was on meds for ADD, which came with their own side effects. She was miserable and it made her mother feel miserable, too. I asked Roxy about how much water her daughter drank on average and she wasn't drinking that much. I asked her to start drinking 16 ounces first thing in the morning and to get her daughter to drink as much as possible.

She agreed. Within a week, she called me overjoyed to tell me that for the first time in her life, her daughter had gone to the bathroom two days in a row. A week later, she told me that her daughter had started to use the bathroom regularly and her stomach aches were gone.

This is not surprising at all.

Now, I don't intend to be gross, but talking about bathroom function is important (and I don't know if you know this, but everyone does it). Our bodies have an endothelial layer that is only one cell layer thick. Reread that: one cell layer thick. It's designed that way because you can pass messages through it and transport what you need, absorbing nutrients along the way. This genius design can become an issue when you don't treat your body properly, though.

If someone is experiencing chronic constipation (and constipation is defined by the National Institutes of Health as having a bowel movement less than three times per week), the toxic waste that is supposed to be on its way out of your body is sitting there, potentially reabsorbing back into your body. What does that look like? Stomach aches, headaches, overburdening your liver, brain fog, sluggishness, hemorrhoids, and a bunch of other things that would make you cringe by just mentioning their name. Why was she constipated? The junk couldn't evacuate because she was nearly perpetually in a constant state of dehydration.

This is not just for kids. I had an adult male client who complained of having to sit on the toilet forever, and even after sitting forever, his guts did not feel great. I recommended that he drastically increase his water intake. Guess what? That issue resolved within two weeks. He was much happier as a result. Okay, bathroom talk over. For now.

What's the point? Drink more water. Like right now. Go ahead, I'll wait.

Improving your bathroom time is not the only reason for you to be flushing your body with water. You've heard that we're 55% (in the elderly) to 75% (infants) water. Don't push this fact aside, relegating it to the dusty spot in your brain where the word riboflavin, mitochondria, metamorphic rocks, and photosynthesis live in the science box in your brain. (You love science, right? Mmm, science.) Dehydration has significant effects not only on your guts, but your mood, and even your ability to think clearly. Many headaches are a side effect of not having adequate water. Being properly hydrated alleviates the burden on your kidneys to get rid of waste products, helps dissolve nutrients and minerals to make them bioavailable, protects body organs, hydrates tissues, regulates body temperature, lubricates joints, and carries nutrients and oxygen to every cell in your body. We are all aware of the fact that you cannot live without water for more than three days, but I want you to be acutely aware of the vital importance that water has to every single cell in your body.

Let me press one more button for you – your vanity. Howard Murad, M.D. is the associate clinical professor of medicine at UCLA, a board certified dermatologist, pharmacist, researcher, and CEO and founder of Murad, Inc. His focus is beyond anti-aging, to the point that he is exploring youth-building and reversing the effects of aging. He proposes that part of the reason we see signs of aging is that our cells cannot properly hold aquatic homeostasis within their membranes, and this leads to the destruction and damage of our cells. His aim is to build youth through supporting and improving cellular integrity, and thus maintaining water homeostasis in every cell. What does this all mean for you? When you're chronically dehydrated, you're going to look old and wrinkly. He has case studies of patients whose wrinkles, fine lines, and acne are going away by employing means of rehydrating cells and building their structural integrity to maintain hydration. Do I have your attention yet? Good. Let's keep going.

What now? You need to know how much water you should be drinking, and that depends on who you are. The Institute of Medicine suggests that on average, adult males need to consume about 3 liters of water daily, whereas females need about 2 liters.[1] If you exercise, you need more. If it's hot, you need more. If you're pregnant or breastfeeding, you'll need more. If you've been sick and lost fluids through diarrhea or vomiting, you'll need more.

Daily Water Intake

Weight (pounds)	Baseline amount (water in oz.)	Exercise: 30 min (water in oz.)	Exercise: 60 min (water in oz.)	Exercise: 90 min (water in oz.)
100	67	79	91	103
125	84	96	108	120
150	101	113	125	137
175	117	129	141	153
200	134	146	158	170
225	151	163	175	187
250	168	180	192	204

The basic rule of thumb is to multiply your weight by 2/3 (0.67) to get your baseline needs, and increase from there depending on other factors (exercise, heat, etc.). For moderate intensity exercise, it is recommended to add about 12 ounces per half hour of exercise.

Did you look at the chart and sigh hopelessly, thinking you'll never be able to drink that much water? Don't panic and don't give up. If you are not accustomed to drinking water on a regular basis, this can seem daunting, but I want to encourage you with this – our bodies can develop a thirst for water. If you have been programming yourself to get by minimally in a chronic state of dehydration, then it will take a little bit to build your thirst, but it can be done easily and without much drama.

How? Drink more, more often. As you practice the habit of drinking water, you will realize that your body will begin to enjoy it and crave water. The start is to get those 16 ounces in before you do anything in the morning. That's basic to rehydrate your body and get it flushed out and ready to go for the day ahead. I drink more than that before I start working out in the morning. I drink while I'm working out, drink after working out, and then carry my water bottle with me throughout the day to make it easily accessible and available whenever I need it. This may sound strange, but the last thing I do before I turn off the light at night is to drink water, too. No, I don't have to get up in the middle of the night to go to the bathroom (although some of my friends argue that waking up before 5:00 a.m. to go swimming is not far off from "the middle of the night", but I digress).

Get into the habit and your body will learn. It will go with the flow (Get it? Water? Flow?), and it doesn't take that long for it to do so. Your recommended daily water intake may seem out of range for you when you start, but it is feasible when you make a plan to get to it. If you're only drinking 30 ounces daily and you need to be somewhere above 120, I recommend that you slowly increase your water intake daily over a period of weeks to help ease yourself into it. These habits and practices are more sustainable and beneficial when you integrate them slowly and naturally into your daily life. Almost anyone can do something crazy for a short time, but my goal for you is to be able to adopt this into your lifestyle so that it is second nature for you. I want you to be able to do this for the rest of your life. My goal is to change your life for the rest of your life, not to shock your body for a few weeks until you're sick of doing it.

What kind of water should you be drinking?

Just as there are different levels of quality in food, cars, wine, and seats at the symphony, there are things that you should take into account about what kind of water you're drinking. You've seen different options as you stroll down the aisle, and you may have wondered how (or why) on earth someone decided to come up with so many different kinds of water. Let's explore a few different options.

As with food, the more that you tamper with water, the more potential there is for screwing it up. Keep this in mind as you think about what is going to work best for you.

Spring water/Artesian wells

The pros? If you have a good clean spring source, this is the best kind of water you can drink. It is filtered through the layers of the earth and contains the trace minerals we need. If you can find a spring near you, by all means, go for it. Check findaspring.com to see what is near you. (I am not advocating for going down to a river somewhere and drinking out of it. This is not safe. When I am referring to spring water, I mean locations where there is a verified, clean, designated spring.) Do your research beforehand, and potentially ask people local to the area for information about it.

The cons? Some people do not live in an area that is close to a natural spring, so this is not necessarily the most convenient option. You also would need to make trips back and forth to the spring to get water, which makes this less convenient than walking into the kitchen and turning on your tap. Some springs are very slow flowing, so you may also have to wait 45 minutes to fill a 5-gallon jug. Know before you go. You also need to verify the safety and cleanliness of a spring before drinking out of it.

Approval rating: A

Tap water

The pros? It's a cheap option. It's easy to access and readily available.

The cons? Depending on where you live, the quality of the water coming out of your tap can vary wildly. If you live on a well, many things can affect the quality of water. The soil that is above your well and the things that runoff onto your land eventually get into your tap and into your body. Are you near a farm that is spraying carcinogenic pesticides like Roundup or near a livestock farm that has biosolid overflow? You may want to rethink drinking it straight. How deep is your well? Do you know if your land has a high presence of naturally occurring chemicals and minerals like arsenic, radon, or uranium? You should also be aware if it has undesirable levels of coliforms (like E. coli!), VOCs (volatile organic compounds), parasites, or nitrates. (To find a lab to test your well, you can contact your state's Health and Human Services department.)

Are you in a place where you get municipal water? In many cities, water is fluoridated and chlorinated. Fluoridation is controversial: many people against fluoridation point to many negative side-effects of this chemical on brain and kidney function. It has been shown to be neurotoxic and to reduce children's IQs. In animal studies, the babies born to mothers who had been exposed to fluoride were hyperactive. After birth, animals that were given fluoride were apathetic, lethargic "couch potatoes", measured by computerized evaluations of behavior.[2] Significant effects have also been shown on thyroid health.

Not every municipality fluoridates their water. There is a movement against doing so in different parts of the United States and the world because of the possible dangers from exposure. You have the right to know what is in your water, and municipal water is tested on a regular basis. If a report is not mailed to you annually, you can contact your local government to find out about your water quality.

Not all tap water is bad. Different locations have different issues, so please educate yourself on your own area to be able to make an informed decision on your own tap water quality.

Approval Rating: C-*

* It could be better or worse. I am accounting for the negative effects of fluoride, and for the remnants of pharmaceuticals that are too small to be filtered out of the water supply. It also makes room for potential baddies in well water, and serious problems like arsenic and elevated levels of lead in some areas.

Water from Plastic Bottles from The Store

The pros? It is potentially cleaner than tap water. It tastes less chloriney.

The cons? It's expensive, wasteful, and the plastic piles up forever and is sure to kill us all. Sometimes the water sources are just from municipal taps anyway. (See above for what that may mean for you.) Read the bottle and check the source.

Exceptions:
Fiji water. It actually comes from Fiji and contains minerals and electrolytes. Unfortunately, it still comes in a plastic bottle, but at least the water is of good quality. Has a pH of about 7.7.

Approval Rating: B- to C-

Household Water Filter Pitchers

The pros? The water tastes better, it's convenient, it's affordable.

The cons? In many of the most popular brands (Brita, Pur, Culligan), the filter creates a significant increase in aluminum (Brita – 33.9% increase, Pur – 46.8% increase, and Culligan – 52.4% increase). Aluminum is significantly linked to Alzheimer's disease[3], and not something you want to add to your diet.

Approval Rating: E*

*Not all household water pitcher filters are this awful. Zero Water filters almost everything and does not add aluminum. The "E" rating is specifically for the popular brands that are mentioned.

Household Gravity Water Filters

The pros? Gravity water filters like Berkey do a great job of filtering out a bunch of stuff: chlorine, chloramine, fluoride, microorganisms, bacteria, heavy metals, and pharmaceuticals. They do not rely on electricity, so in an emergency, you can have very clean water. They are reasonably easy to transport and set up.

The cons? Depending on what you get, they can verge on being somewhat gigantic. That's not so much of a problem if you have a McMansion, but if your house is lacking space, you may not want a giant quasi-cylindrical statuette among your accoutrements. That's up to you, though.

Approval Rating: A- (A+ if you have a McMansion)

Distilled Water

The pros? It's really clean.

The cons? The absence of minerals in distilled water are going to strip your body and send you to an early grave. You need electrolytes like sodium, potassium, chloride, and magnesium for your heart to function well. Stripping your body of these minerals can lead to a host of problems including osteoporosis, osteoarthritis, hypothyroidism, hypertension, coronary artery disease, and premature aging. It's also acidic, which many believe is the environment in which disease thrives.

Approval Rating: D

Water Filters that Adjust pH Levels

The pros? Having a machine that can change the pH of water is kind of cool, like you are some kind of groovy science magician. Some people claim that with water of extremely high pH levels, you can immediately cure headaches, migraines, etc.

The cons? There is not much use for acidic water. Some people advocate for water with a higher alkaline pH level, suggesting that it is good for your body because disease cannot live in an alkaline environment. People who think that alkaline water is useless junk say so because they point out that the human body always seeks homeostasis – which means if you introduce an alkaline substance, it will increase acid production to counterbalance it. (Ironic, since that is the thing you were trying to get away from.) Machines that adjust pH levels are also quite expensive and do not filter out heavy metals, chlorine, pharmaceuticals, and whatever else is left from municipal (or well) water sources.

Approval Rating: D

Reverse Osmosis Water

The pros? It's really clean. It can be fitted to your tap to purify your water of chlorine, fluoride (you need to get a specific filter for this), pharmaceuticals, lead, asbestos, iron, mercury, parasitical water-borne cysts, and a bunch of other junk that you don't want in your body. The water tastes significantly better when filtered through reverse osmosis.

The cons? It strips minerals, too. This is the same problem as distilled water. (See: early grave.) It usually has a storage tank, which can be dicey for some people if they are low on space. Most people get around this by housing it under their sink (or by finding creative ways up from the basement).

Approval Rating: D

Reverse Osmosis Water with Remineralization

The pros? It's super clean, and tastes great. It contains beneficial minerals, so you're not having your body leached of what you need to function properly. It is relatively easy to set up. Some companies offer a tube that the reverse osmosis water runs through, where it will pick up minerals. Another option is to get remineralization drops.

The cons? Once you are used to the taste of this water, you will absolutely become a water snob. You will watch your friends fill up their water bottles at the drinking fountain at the gym, shake your head sadly, and know in your heart that you could only succumb to that if you were near literally dying of thirst, since now with your highly sensitive palate, you will sense that you are drinking straight from the swimming pool If you have a remineralization tube, it's difficult to know precisely when the mineral content is diminished. You need to make a note of when you ought to change it. If you are using remineralization drops, it is difficult to know exactly how much you should be adding to water. If your water bottle is partially filled, how do you reconcile the difference exactly when you want to fill it? Is it possible to do? Absolutely. Is it the most convenient thing? Not really.

Approval Rating: A- (remineralization tube)/B+ (remineralization drops)

What should I drink out of?

It is so important for you to get a water bottle and to bring it with you throughout the day so that you can drink from it whenever the mood arises. There are several different options on the market. I'll start with the best options first.

Stainless Steel Water Bottles

These are a great option because they can be sterilized, do not leach, and do not break. If you get a good double-walled water bottle, you can keep a steady temperature even in extreme conditions. The negatives are that some people complain that they don't prefer the taste of water when drinking out of stainless steel. Stainless steel water bottles won't break, but if you're a little rough on them, they can dent. Extra bonus: you look cool and sort of tough when you accessorize with it.

Glass Water Bottles

Maybe it's just me, but water tastes the best out of glass. Glass can be sterilized, and it won't leach. Some glass water bottles have rubbery sleeves that help prevent breakage, but when it comes down to it, it's still glass and has the potential for breaking. One more negative: a full glass water bottle sinks in the pool when your friends accidentally knock it in (don't tell the lifeguard you have one, either).

Ceramic Water Bottles

Ceramic water bottles are not very popular (yet?) because although they are not plastic (bonus), they have a few drawbacks: they're heavy, they're breakable, many don't have good seals on their closing mechanisms (i.e., a cork), and the cracks in the glazing on the insides can hold bacteria. The glazing material may also be less than optimal for health and you may tire of people asking you why you're drinking out of a vase.

Plastic Water Bottles

Can I be absolutely honest? They're junk. Don't drink out of them. While it's true that they don't (usually) break, they do leach, and because of that, you don't want to pour in very hot water. That puts a damper on cleaning it well. The plastic from disposable water bottles is even worse.

Even if your bottle says BPA free, it can still leach other chemicals. I have a sneaking suspicion that BPA-free labeling is going to end up like how "sugar-free" did (that would be how we landed in a pile of aspartame with leukemia and lymphoma).

Action Steps

Over these next two weeks, I want to encourage you to bump up your water intake. Before anything else, drink 16 ounces of water in the morning to get things going in the right direction. If you are far from your goal of how much you ought to be drinking, make a plan. Take inventory of where you are right now and map it out. Write it down in a notebook, track it on an app, envision me standing on your shoulder whispering in your ear, use a dot planner, and/or call your mother and tell her to keep you accountable, whatever works. You can do this. Now pull up your big girl panties (or manly boy boxers) and get after it.

Chapter 3:
Food You Should Eat

Two-week goal: Experiment in improving one or more areas within the food categories mentioned in this chapter.

Food seems like it is the most controversial, confusing, and biggest topic regarding health. One news article tells of the wonders of dairy, while another warns us that dairy will bring us to a mucousy and early death. Some experts tell us that whole grains and wheat are part of our balanced diet, while others tell us that gluten is the source of all evil and bodily inflammation. Some will say that you ought to eat low fat foods to be in optimal health, while another boasts about the wonders of good fats and how they help our brains to function well. If it sounds confusing, you're not alone. I get questions about food more than any other subject, and I want to break that down for you and make it easy. I have a very simple philosophy when it comes to eating: If God didn't make it, don't eat it. (Do not eat lab created inventions, man-made whims, or fantastical science experiments.) The reverse is mostly true, but it depends on your own constitution, and that is: if God made it, you can probably eat it.

In this chapter, I will take a category or types of food, give you a little bit of the controversy surrounding it, and try to simplify it and educate you so that you can make the best choices for yourself and for your family.

Dairy

Let's begin at the beginning. As a baby, you very likely drank some form of milk or formula pretending to imitate milk. You likely grew up eating all forms of dairy (unless perhaps you have an intolerance or an allergy), and even now you probably consume a few servings of dairy each day. The dairy industry in the United States is enormous. To get an idea of just exactly what "enormous" looks like, the projection for 2016 for the dairy industry in just the United States had market shares around $56.8 billion. You'd have a difficult time ignoring an industry with that kind of weight in the world.

With an influence that strong, you are going to hear a lot of positive things about dairy, simply because the industry is so vast, has so much money, and is a significant portion of the nation's entire economy. This is not to say that dairy is inherently good or bad, but critical thinking will lead you to understand that the voice against dairy will not have as strong of an influence as the pro-dairy side.

With that being said, here are some of the arguments surrounding dairy:

1. Dairy is only meant for baby cows, not for human consumption. It is inherently bad and should not be a human food.

Dairy certainly is meant for baby cows. Cows are mammals and baby mammals drink milk. I don't think anyone will disagree with that. Is dairy for you? That's a trickier question.

Let's start with the opposite – who should not be drinking dairy?

If you are allergic or intolerant to dairy, you will obviously raise your hand and excuse yourself from the dairy party. If you are sensitive to some dairy, then you should take care in what you consume. Have you ever spoken with someone who can eat some forms of dairy but not others?

Maybe they can have yogurt and certain cheeses, but not straight milk. Have you ever thought about why this might be?

A large majority of people who say that they can have some forms of dairy but not another usually say that they can digest cultured dairy (like yogurt and cheese). This is because of the reintroduction of enzymes that help break down the milk for digestion. It is easier to digest food that already contains enzymes. Your body doesn't have to work quite as hard to contribute their own to the digestive process.

I personally do not believe that all dairy is inherently evil, but I do think that there are a lot of people who are sensitive to it but are not aware of it because they have never removed it from their diets for long enough to experience a positive reaction without it. Many of my clients who experiment with removing dairy from their diets for 3-6 weeks report positive results: they no longer have any congestion, they are less mucousy overall, they experience less gas, and they have a better time on the toilet.

You should also consider your genetic makeup. If your ancestors traditionally did not consume dairy products, it may be wiser to avoid it, or at least experiment within your own body as to how you react without it. If your ancestors are from the Emmental region of Switzerland, your DNA is more likely to support some serious cheese eating. Just because a food is readily available and promoted to you does not mean that it is beneficial for you to consume it.

I encourage many of my clients to give themselves the gift of understanding how their body functions with or without dairy. It is a knowledge that many will not explore for themselves (because living without a nice smoked gouda seems kind of like a pointless life to some), but if you are brave and inclined to learn about yourself and what your body needs and wants, I implore you to remove it for a time and to listen to your body. There is only knowledge and understanding to be gained and three weeks without your beloved cheese is sure to earn you a patch for the Difficult Trials of Life on your Girl Scout uniform and undoubtedly make you more able to identify with the suffering of the world.

2. Low fat dairy is the best because you don't want to gain extra weight by drinking full-fat milk or consuming full-fat dairy products.

I'm just going to come out and directly say that this makes me cringe. If you were alive in the 80s and 90s, you were inundated and powerfully brainwashed with the rhetoric of low-fat and the benefits we are sure to gain from it.

Have you looked around lately? How is that working out for us?

I'll let the facts speak for us. We're fatter than ever. It's not working. In fact, studies show the opposite is true.[4] People who ate full-fat dairy are leaner than those who eat skim, non-fat, or low-fat dairy. Maybe your knee jerk reaction is to say that that must be because people who are skinny just eat whatever they want and don't care. They're just built differently. This is not the case. The chicken came before the egg – full fat dairy corresponds to being leaner because of its consumption; low fat dairy corresponds to a higher risk of central obesity. Let me put it to you like this: if you want to be fat, eat low-fat dairy. If you want to stand a chance to be leaner, eat full fat. (I know it seems ironic, but that's because you still believe that fat makes you fat. Fat doesn't make you fat. Sugar makes you fat. Tattoo that on the inside of your brain.)

The dairy industry is not only filthy stinking rich, but they are also geniuses. They pump up cows with growth hormones like rBST (which get passed on to you, unfortunately) to increase milk production (with an added bonus of screwing up your endocrine system and sending your little girls into puberty early – that's exactly what you don't need). From that single output they make myriads of products to sell to you: cheese, butter, cream, yogurt, etc. Talk about creativity and resourcefulness! Even the milk is broken up into different products. You can get whole milk, 2% milk, ½ % milk, and skim or non-fat milk. If you allow whole non-homogenized milk to separate into cream solids and milk, you can make several different products – the cream can be skimmed off of the top to make cream or butter, and the rest can be sold as different varieties of milk. That's how you get to make good money – one source and many products equals many streams of revenue coming in.

Thus, it is a financial advantage to convince people of the usefulness of skim milk and to create a demand for it. Please don't fall for it. If you're going to consume dairy, make sure it is full-fat. Regarding dairy quality, you want to first find milk or dairy products from grass-fed cows, then secondly organic, and in third and final place is conventional growth-hormone, antibiotic-laden, sad, enzyme-free milk.

Reflect back – the closer the state the milk is to its original is how you want to eat. What does that mean for low-fat dairy? It means that if you're going to eat it at all, go for full-fat, just how the cows are delivering it to you.

3. Raw/fresh milk is dangerous, and pasteurized milk is the best invention since sliced bread.

This is an argument that could start small wars in places. Here's the deal. The entire world drank unpasteurized milk for a few thousand plus years until Louis Pasteur figured he should try this new way in 1864. I wholeheartedly agree that if you are going to be a large scale dairy farmer who doesn't know their herd, you inherently must use pasteurization to keep things clean and good for your customers. I'm going to shock some of you, so hold on tight – I do not believe that this is the best way to consume milk, but it is the best and safest way to sell milk.

If you are a family with one cow in your backyard, you will know the health of your little Bessie, and you will take care to be clean and careful. That is because you are personally involved in drinking the milk and caring for an animal that means something to you and your family. When things move to a large scale operation, you must hire people to take care of your animals. That becomes their job, and not necessarily their passion. It does not nourish their body or that of their family. They are removed from the process by a level. Even with the world's best micromanager, you still may have things slip out from under your control. You can't run a business that is a liability waiting to happen, so you must take precautionary steps to protect yourself. That is where pasteurization comes in, and where it rightly should come in.

Unfortunately, we are missing out on quality milk as a result of our mass production. Fresh milk contains enzymes that help with digestion that are killed off through the process of pasteurization. (It's almost like they were put there on purpose. Huh.) Once you've smelled it, you'll never forget the smell of putrid pasteurized milk that went bad and was sitting in a small puddle in the bottom of a milk jug in the recycling bin. It's absolutely horrific. Do you know what happens when you leave raw milk out on the counter? It turns to cheese - that you could really eat and not gag from the scent. If you've never tasted raw milk, it tastes about the same as pasteurized, but a little sweeter.

Small scale farming is not the way of the mega-billion-dollar dairy industry, however, so it is not in their best interest to support such things. It is in their best interest to convince you of the near-certain death that awaits you with your first sip of guaranteed E. coli-laden raw milk. It is in their best interest for you not to be aware that of the 48,000,000 food borne illnesses annually, 42 are a result of raw milk. Your great-grandmother would be shocked at your reckless behavior for even thinking to do such a thing. Wait.

Nutrients in raw milk (like probiotics, Vitamin D, and immunoglobulins) help boost the immune system and actually reduce allergies. The healthy saturated fats and omega-3s in raw milk are remedies for eczema, acne, and skin issues through topical use or ingestion. (You already knew that European soap makers use milk in their specialty soaps, right?) One serving of raw milk loads you up with magnesium, calcium, and potassium. It contains the fat soluble vitamins like Vitamin A, D, and K2, supporting your brain health, bone density, and hormone levels. The fatty acids, CLA, and omega-3s in raw grass-fed milk reduce inflammation, help your body deal with stress, and even support your metabolism. Pasteurization reduces or destroys the following nutrients in milk: Vitamin A, C, E, iron, zinc, B-complex, enzymes, calcium, immunoglobulins, and even denatures whey protein.

Many states do not allow you to directly purchase raw milk (I wonder who wanted that to happen), but you can do things like purchase a share in a cow and then go pick up your own milk, and pay your farmer for the care of the animal. If you decide to participate in a cow-share, I encourage you to get to know your farmer and how they treat the cows beforehand. Ask how often they are out to pasture, how much land they're able to graze on, what they eat in the winter, how many cows are in their herd, and how they deal with sickness in their animals. You will learn more than you ever thought you could from your local small-scale dairy farmer. They are exceptionally tough and have earned my respect. They are working with the land and healing the soil and they get my highest stamp of approval.

If you're going to consume dairy at all, here's the quick list (best to worst):

1. Local, raw, non-homogenized, grass-fed, pastured dairy
2. Grass-fed dairy (full-fat is best)
3. Organic dairy (full-fat is best)
4. Conventional full-fat dairy
5. Conventional low-fat dairy

Meat

The controversy around meat consumption usually comes mainly from a vegetarian or vegan perspective, or from a cultural or religious perspective from avoiding a certain animal (or animals). Within the vegetarian or vegan thought are at least two reasons for advocating against eating meat: 1) meat is inherently unhealthy and you shouldn't eat it, and 2) the way that animals are treated for consumption is so horrifying that it is wrong to support an industry that practices business in that unethical manner. Within the religious or cultural perspectives, certain foods are avoided because they are considered unclean or because they are holy or sacred, neither of which would be appropriate for consumption.

Should you eat meat? It really is an individual choice and depends on how your body responds to meat or lack of it (and what kind), but let me give you why you may or may not want to consider doing so.

If you have a conviction or a religious or cultural belief to not eat meat (or certain types of meat), I will not attempt to convince you otherwise. Could you be missing out on certain things as a result? Possibly, but I would think that living in line with your beliefs will help you sleep better at night a lot more than the consumption of a barbecue chicken sandwich eaten under duress would.

One of the reasons that you would not want to eat meat (or very much of it) would be if your ancestors did not eat it. You share the DNA that your great-great-great grandfather had, and that of his great-great-great grandfather. I believe that certain things resonate with your body and your cells. There is something to be said about eating in a traditional manner, based on the areas of the globe that your DNA hailed from. Have you ever felt emotionally and physically nourished from eating a comfort food from your own personal lineage? It's in your genes. You're a new soul, but the genes in your body have been around for a very long time.

Another reason that you may want to forgo meat for a time is if you are not able to purchase high-quality, ethically and properly raised and slaughtered meats. The old adage "you are what you eat" is truer than we thought. Consuming an animal that lived in slummy conditions, not eating a natural diet, cranked up on hormones, crammed in small spaces, and mistreated by handlers is an animal that will have lived a life full of stress and ill-health. You're absorbing that into your own body when you consume it. Stress in an animal alters the protein composition, vitamin content, and minerals. If purchasing a higher quality meat is difficult because of budget, I would advocate for spending money on the best you can afford while balancing out the rest in a more vegetarian manner. Whenever I go out to eat and I am not familiar with the meat quality, I purposely choose to eat in a vegetarian way.

There are a few studies out there like the *China Study* (by Dr. T. Collin Campbell) that suggest that eating a plant-based diet will help you avoid cancer, but the research has been discredited and is under significant scrutiny for being a prime example of bad science, lacking credibility. The claims that Campbell made in his book were not supported by the raw data, and some information was cherry picked and blatantly ignored because it did not fit with his preconceived notion and agenda for a vegan lifestyle. This is lamentable, but reminds us of the importance of good science and drawing proper correlations and conclusions from data.

The other popular outlet for this theology comes from the documentary, *Forks Over Knives*. Unfortunately, the filmmakers relied heavily on the conclusions of Campbell to set their scene. In watching this film, the comparison of what was eaten before switching to a plant-based diet is not made. I would think that anyone would see an improvement in their biometrics if they were originally addicted to fast food, sugar, processed foods, and beer. What were the participants eating? Were they eating grass-fed meats? Were they eating pastured and humanely raised chicken and organic local vegetables? The information is lacking, and I have a suspicion that it was purposely omitted.

On the other side of the coin, there are some good reasons to eat meat. Most traditional cultures do consume meat, but in varying types because of climate and location (thus, not much reindeer meat in Fiji or saltwater clams in western Mongolia). Look to your heritage and consider what was eaten for thousands of years as you consider whether or not this is optimal for you.

Meat contains significant sources of protein, and all of the amino acids, iron, selenium, zinc, and vitamins like A, D, and B. If you are a vegetarian, you've likely heard someone ask you how your Vitamin B12 levels are – it is one of the major concerns within a vegetarian diet because it is not present in plant foods. Vitamin B12 is responsible for supporting your nerves, brain, and creating red blood cells, giving you clear mental function, and energy. The nutrients in meat are also quickly and readily bioavailable, making it possible for your body to get what it needs rapidly.

I experienced the wonders of this several years ago. I had a failed pregnancy and had to deliver my baby at about 20 weeks' gestation. I was whisked off to the very last room down a long hallway in the labor and delivery wing of the hospital and was induced to have contractions. It took about ten hours for me to deliver my tiny baby, but once he was born, the doctor, midwife, and nurses began to become concerned because the placenta was not cooperating and making its grand exit. All at once, my blood pressure dropped dangerously low and I lost consciousness and turned grey. The next thing I knew, I was on a gurney with my doctor and the nurses running down a hallway into an operating room. They told me to count down from ten, but I don't remember even hitting eight. I woke up later to find myself back in my room, recovering. I had a hard time walking after that – it felt like when you have the flu and your legs burn from walking up the stairs, your breathing is labored, and doing anything except laying down takes your breath away and exhausts you. I was anemic and my usual peppy self was reduced to choosing fun activities like either sleeping on the couch or sleeping in a bed because I didn't have the energy to do challenging things like walk to the kitchen and sit up at the table.

I researched sources of iron and found a very high (albeit disgusting) one – beef liver. I did not grow up eating organ meats, and the thought of them was repulsive, but I had to suck it up and deal with it because of what it was going to be able to provide for my body. I insisted that I was going to cook it, so in order to accommodate me, my mother dragged a chair into the kitchen and put it in front of the stove so I could do it. I was so pathetically weak that I couldn't stand up long enough by myself to cook a piece of meat. I used a recipe that promised you would love liver if you ate it this way, but after one bite, I realized this would never be the case. I ate an entire serving of that disgusting meat, half of the time swallowing it whole like vitamins, medicinally, but hoping that it would make me feel better. It did. Within about twelve hours, I was able to walk from room to room. I ate it again the following day and noticed another marked improvement, feeling a great deal more energy than I had since before the delivery. I ate it once more for the last time, and almost felt human again. It was powerfully bioavailable, and made a huge difference in my recovery.

Besides these important nutrients, animal foods uniquely contain creatine (which forms an energy reserve in muscles), carnosine (an antioxidant that protects against many degenerative processes), DHA, and EPA (active forms of omega-3s. ALA is the plant form of omega-3s, but the body is inefficient at converting it to an active form). All of these nutrients are only found in animal products.

There are a few types of meat that you will want to avoid inherently – those are processed meats that contain funky sodiums: sodium nitrate and sodium nitrite. These are found in lunch meats, bacon, bologna, corned beef, hot dogs, sausages, canned meats, and cured meats. Before you throw down this book angrily for seemingly suggesting that you avoid bacon, I want to point out to you that these are just the locations where you're likely to find these bad guys. Not all bacons, bologna, sausages, and hot dogs contain them, but you have to seek out the clean ones. And you really ought to do so, because your risk for pancreatic cancer increases dramatically from the consumption of these processed meats.[5] There is also a link to brain tumors and non-Hodgkin lymphoma (blood cancer) with the consumption of sodium nitrates and sodium nitrites.[6] Clean bacon is better than no bacon, right?

Meat Labels

Be aware of different labels as you purchase meat. The word "natural" means nothing. There is no regulation that decides what this can or cannot mean. Arsenic and dog poop are natural. This does not influence me to eat either one. Sometimes there will be a label on poultry highlighting the fact that they are not using hormones for their chickens, turkeys, or other birds. They're not allowed to. The USDA prohibits the use of hormones for poultry, so they're bragging about something that is law anyway. Do not be impressed. "Amish" chicken is also an unimpressive label. It means nothing. If a company is sourcing some chicken from an Amish farm, that may be fine, but it doesn't mean that they are free-ranging amongst children dressed in black and white clothing, running barefoot in green meadows, waving to the grandma with her quilt on the buggy going by. You totally picture that, though, and it's great for marketing. "Vegetarian fed" is another label that sounds like it would be a good thing, but really isn't. If they are guaranteeing that chicken is "vegetarian fed", what that likely means is that the chickens are eating corn and soy and not out to pasture eating bugs and grass, like they're supposed to. My chickens are not "vegetarian fed" – they run around in the backyard and eat worms, bugs, spiders, and I am happy that they do so. That's what they're supposed to do. "Cage free" seems like it is also a good thing, and it's better than being in a cage, but not by much if it means that animals are housed in long, windowless, corrugated metal buildings, never allowed to see the light of day and stepping all over each other from crowding.

If you have a local farmer's market, you may find quality meat there. Ask your farmer if the animals are out on pasture, if they are given antibiotics or hormones, what they eat, and where their farm is. Sometimes farmers farm in an organic and land-conscious way, but do not go through the expensive and lengthy process to get certified as such. It may be that you're getting exactly what you want without a label, so it's worth it to ask. Most farmers are not allowed to butcher their own meat, so you may also want to ask about their processing.

The labels that you want to look for are the following:

1. "Grass fed" is a term that is usually applied to beef. Bison are inherently grass fed because they won't eat anything else (although some farmers have tried). Cows are supposed to eat grass. They are not supposed to eat corn or anything else. It is damaging to their digestive systems to do so, and causes gastrointestinal stress and illness. This is a label worth paying extra for. Grass fed meats have a higher omega 3 count, and are leaner. If you're eating grass fed meat, it must have been out to pasture which means it was able to express its natural lifestyle. Stress in an animal is reduced, and that translates into the meat, which translates into your own body. Joel Salatin, a famous author, farmer, public speaker, (one of my heroes) and real food advocate calls this the "pigness of the pig" – allowing animals to do exactly what they are meant to do in the proper environment and in harmony with the land. This healthy balance benefits the animal, the earth, and all of humanity.
2. "Free range" or "pastured" means something different than "cage free". Free range means that they must have access to going outside, and pastured means that they get to go out to pasture. Cage free means neither one of those things. Look for "pastured" or "free range" on your poultry.
3. "Wild caught" is the preferred label for fish. Factory farmed fish are the ones with the genetic modification and experimentation going on, and we have not seen any long-term studies proving that those are safe for human consumption.

If you are going to eat meat, here are the healthiest to least healthy alternatives:

1. Grass-fed, local beef/bison/etc.; free-range and pastured poultry (non-soy diet); wild-caught fish
2. Organic beef, poultry, pork, lamb, etc.

3. Conventional feedlot beef, poultry, pork, etc., and factory farmed fish.

Produce

Thankfully there is not a lot of controversy over people eating vegetables and fruit (there is perhaps a question regarding quantity of fruit because of sugar, but other than that, I do not know many who have problems with people eating their veggies). The recurring question regarding produce is usually geared at organic versus conventionally grown, and if either matter, or if fresh, canned, or frozen veggies and fruits are best.

There is a wide spectrum of belief regarding eating produce organically or not. If you are on an impossible budget, I would recommend you eat fruits and veggies and not fall apart over the labeling. If your budget has some flexibility or if you are able to arrange things to spend a little more, there is a handy list called the "Dirty Dozen" and the "Clean Fifteen" put out by the Environmental Working Group (find them at ewg.org). Each year they test myriads of fruits and veggies to let you know which have the highest and lowest pesticide load and rank them. This is very helpful because if you are not able to purchase everything organically, you at least have a guide to purchase the most toxic things organically, avoiding over 90% of pesticides by doing so.

The guide changes annually, but almost every year that I have been paying attention, strawberries and apples are near the top. They have found that one apple can have 47 different pesticides on it. Because you eat the entire surface area almost every time you eat a strawberry, it is pretty important to purchase these organically if you are able. If you or your child suffers from ADD or ADHD, these are things you want to especially avoid because of the connection to worsening that condition[7]. You can go to their website and download (for free) a PDF guide of the current year's list.

Here is this year's worst of the worst produce for pesticide load in order from top baddy down.

The Dirty Dozen (2017)

1	Strawberries
2	Spinach
3	Nectarines
4	Apples
5	Peaches
6	Pears
7	Cherries
8	Grapes
9	Celery
10	Tomatoes
11	Sweet bell peppers
12	Potatoes

If you have the chance to purchase these twelve organically, please do so. You can avoid the most pesticides in your body this way.

The Clean Fifteen are the fifteen fruits and veggies with the least pesticide content, allowing for a space in your budget where you can feel a little more comfortable purchasing conventionally grown produce. Some people feel inclined to purchase all of their produce organically, and if that is what you want, by all means, do so. These are the safest options to purchase conventionally if your budget requires creativity.

As far as nutritional content, fresh (and local – like your backyard, if you can) veggies are usually the highest, followed by frozen vegetables and fruits, with canned fruits and vegetables falling in last. Canned vegetables and fruits (and canned goods in general) are usually in aluminum cans, which increases your aluminum exposure and your risk of Alzheimer's. Unfortunately, most canned products also have BPA sprayed onto the insides of the can and you have to look specifically for labels telling you otherwise. Having a side of BPA with your green beans is never recommended.

Clean Fifteen (2017)

1	Sweet corn
2	Avocados
3	Pineapples
4	Cabbage
5	Onions
6	Sweet peas (frozen)
7	Papayas
8	Asparagus
9	Mangoes
10	Eggplant
11	Honeydew melon
12	Kiwi
13	Cantaloupe
14	Cauliflower
15	Grapefruit

Eggs

Eggs are a food near and dear to me because I am the proud owner and caretaker of a dozen(ish) laying hens. If I could only have one kind of animal for the rest of my life, it would be chickens. They know the way to my heart through providing me a delicious fresh breakfast (cooked in grass-fed butter on a cast iron pan) every morning.

Chickens are funny little creatures, and if you aren't very familiar with them, you may be surprised that they actually each have their own little personalities. The question that most people have regarding eggs is what is best to buy and what they should be looking out for.

Let me explain a few things about chickens and eggs because I have heard some comments that made me realize that perhaps the mystery of chickens and egg laying is not exceptionally common knowledge, and if you are armed with this, you may be able to make more conscientious and educated decisions regarding your egg consumption.

I once told a vegan friend that I owned chickens for eggs and she commented that the chickens must be upset with me for taking their babies every morning. I looked at her in a perplexed manner and explained that I only had hens. She didn't know what this explanation had to do with anything until I told her about the laying cycle of chickens. Forgive me if you know this already, but I need to just get it out there. Hens lay eggs. Female humans have eggs, too. Just like female humans do not need any males to produce an egg, hens do not need a rooster to produce their eggs. But just as female humans need a male to fertilize their egg to reproduce, so too a hen needs a rooster to reproduce. Hens are on an ovulatory cycle of about once a day or once every other day. Women are on a cycle that typically lasts about a month. Eggs laid by hens without a rooster fertilizing them (i.e., the eggs in your grocery store and at your farmer's market) do not contain embryonic baby chickens. If you sit on them and keep them warm, they will not turn into chicks. They are not fertilized. They are breakfast.

Eggs come in different colors. It is very popular to think that brown eggs are much healthier than white eggs, I mean, after all, isn't brown (wheat) bread healthier than white? And isn't brown rice better than white rice? And isn't chocolate better than vanilla? But this is not inherently the case for eggs. Ready for this? The breed of chicken determines what color egg they lay. I have an Araucana chicken (named Ari) who lays blue-grey eggs. Sweetie (my favorite chicken) is a White Rock who lays brown eggs. They are all in relatively the same health condition (most of the time), they all get to go out to pasture and peck bugs, worms, and grass, and they all eat the same feed mix and kitchen scraps. The exterior color of their egg is not important. What's inside is what counts (just like your mother always told you).

What is important for your eggs is to source them from a farm or a home that allows for the "chickenness of the chicken" (as Joel Salatin would say). It is not natural or optimal for chickens to be stacked in cages, pooping on each other's heads, never allowed to walk outside and act in a way that is perfectly normal for them. It is not optimal for chickens to be crammed into overpopulated places and treated only as objects of revenue. (And to be sure, I'm not against making profit for selling eggs – I do it when I can, but my animals are treated humanely and allowed to live a normal chicken life.) The life of an animal will reflect into what it produces for you, and you will absorb whatever it is that they did. I know that this sounds strange or hocus pocus at first, but in thinking critically about what stress and living in a way that is incongruent to our nature does to humans, we are remiss to overlook how such things affect an animal's life, and in so doing, affect our own. (My quick meat motto: eat animals that had happy, normal lives.) Our stress is stored in our bodies, and in those of animals also.

Have you seen pictures of eggs in baskets laying out on counters? Did you ever wonder why they were not in the refrigerator? The eggs that you get from the store have been washed in a bleach-water solution (let's get real – chickens are not exceptionally pristine animals), which also washes off a natural protective barrier. Once that happens, eggs need to be refrigerated. (Just imagine all of those eggs being laid in the summer months. "Oh no! These fresh eggs have been sitting in the nesting box for two hours! They've gone bad!" That's not a thing.) If you have backyard hens or access to unwashed eggs, you can leave your eggs out on the counter (or wash them and put them in the fridge).

So what are some qualities to look for in a good egg? Referring back to the basic way of thinking about how you ought to eat – that is, eating as close to nature and in as close to the original state as possible – you would want to find an egg that came from a chicken that was allowed to behave like a chicken. That looks like (if you need to go label hunting) "pastured" or "free range". "Cage free" is a step down from that because it doesn't mean that they get to go outside, it just means that they get to live their lives outside of a cage. "Organic" eggs mean that the chickens had access to organic feed, which is great, but if you want a step up from that, choose a farmer who is not feeding his or her chickens soy (you don't need any more estrogenic compounds in your body than you already have – and that's what soy is). How do you know what the chickens are eating? Call and ask the farm. And like with anything else, choosing something that is more local is going to give you a fresher product while cutting down on food miles and supporting your local economy.

Best to worst – eggs:

1. Eggs from your happy chickens in your backyard or your local farm that are allowed to run around and peck bugs and grass, who eat an organic, soy-free feed.
2. "Pastured" or "free range" organic eggs.
3. "Cage free" eggs (organic is better).
4. Bleach-washed, cooped up, poopy-headed conventional chicken eggs.

Breads, Wheat, and Carbs

Boule, challah, stollen, naan, brioche, focaccia, chapati, tortillas, pasta – we love you. We can't really help it, with all the deliciousness going on, who could blame us? (Besides the Paleo, Whole 30, and the Atkins people, I mean.) The controversy here is whether or not we ought to be eating it at all, and if we should be, what kind is best?

If you have a wheat allergy or a condition like Crohn's or celiac disease, or a non-celiac gluten sensitivity, you've got to find other options besides glutinous carbohydrates in order to make your body happy. This is true for many people suffering from other conditions like PCOS (poly-cystic ovarian syndrome), rheumatoid arthritis, Hashimoto's, Graves' disease (or any autoimmune thyroid disease), liver disease, and more as so many things are related to gluten sensitivity and inflammation.

If you've ever considered it, there are some positives for ditching gluten (even if you do it as an experiment for 3-6 weeks). I have a female client in her 50s who has been suffering from RA for the last sixteen years. This amazing woman had gone through times of complete debilitation, pain, and an inability on some days to even get out of bed. She gave up gluten (and started taking curcumin) as an experiment. After a very short time (within 2-4 weeks), she came back to report how she was doing. She walked in to our meeting, excited, happy, and glowing. She walked up to me and gave me a hug and said, "Watch this!" She raised her arms up over her head, completely straight, then bent down into a squat and stood back up. She had not been able to do that for a decade and a half. This was the summer time and it was the first time she had been able to garden in over fifteen years. Her family didn't know what to do with her, she was carrying loads of mulch back and forth from her driveway to her backyard, yanking weeds, and enjoying the dirt. She was living her life the way that she wanted to for the first time in a very long time. She had energy and she felt great. It was not long after that she went in for an appointment with her rheumatologist, who declared that she was officially in remission and for her to keep up whatever it was she was doing.

She knows what her body wants and how it functions optimally now. A few months after this breakthrough, she went to a restaurant and tried some breadsticks. She was sick in bed and in pain for the rest of the weekend. She called me and told me she absolutely knew what her body wanted and how to listen to it now. This is the real success. Having the ability to understand what your body wants and to be able to give it what it needs is the key to living healthy.

A male client cut all gluten and grains for three weeks and then lost 20 pounds in 35 days. In fact, every one of my clients who chose to forgo gluten for even a few weeks lost weight. (I also make sure that they are eating real, whole foods during that time.) If this is one of your goals, it is worth trying. Pay attention to your body in that time. Note how you feel in mental clarity, your energy levels, how your digestive system is responding to the change, your sleep, and your weight.

The only caution on this is with some sprinting athletes, because you will switch from glucose to ketones when you cut gluten (and grains), your sprinting times may suffer. Distance athletes may not have the same problem, however, and some ultra-marathoners swear that going paleo and gluten-free is the way to go. If you are an athlete, take caution and experiment with how your body responds to removing gluten if you choose to do so.

If you are not interested (or do not do well) in avoiding gluten or grains, you should be aware of the healthiest versions so you can make the best decisions for your body.

The wheat and the grains that we commonly eat today are much more complicated than those of thousands of years ago. Are you ready for some science? Scientists have been interested in mapping various genomes (genomes are the complete set of genes or genetic material present in a cell or organism – it contains all of the information needed to build that organism and allow it to grow and develop). Today's wheat is a hexaploid species. That means its genome contains six copies of each of its seven chromosomes. Its constituent number of paired DNA bases (nucleotides) is so massive that it is five times the amount of the DNA in the human genome. It contains 42 chromosomes (6 sets of the seven chromosomes), whereas the human genome is a diploid – it contains 23 pairs of chromosomes (2 of each), to give us 46 chromosomes. Why is that complicated and what does that have to do with anything?

Have you heard of "ancient grains"? Many companies are jumping on the health food bus by promoting "ancient grains" like teff, amaranth, spelt, emmer, einkorn, sorghum, millet, and others. Einkorn is a diploid species (two chromosomes each) and emmer is a tetraploid (four sets). Ancient grains are usually thought of as more nutritious than the modern grains, containing more antioxidants, vitamins, minerals, and protein. The modern grains also have a higher amount of gluten and starch which give them a higher glycemic index (which means they will spike your blood sugar higher). The modern wheat is a more complex species, which may be why it causes trouble for so many. The modern wheat has also been modified to withstand a certain pesticide load, which is genius for wheat farming and output, but may not be the very best thing nutritionally for the consumer.

One way to increase the ability for your body to digest and absorb minerals and vitamins within a grain is to use it in its sprouted form. Ezekiel bread is an example of a sprouted bread. A wheat berry is essentially a seed, and when it is sprouted, the tiny sprout breaks through the bran (imagine the elementary school experiment of a bean in a plastic bag with a wet paper towel). A sprouted grain increases the B vitamins in a grain, along with folate, fiber, and vitamin C. It also increases essential amino acids, which are not usually present in grains. Another benefit of sprouted grains is that they are potentially less allergenic than their unsprouted counterparts. Sprouting decreases gluten proteins significantly, which is another component of making digestion easier.

You probably have heard the health gurus preaching at you to avoid white flour (and white sugar) – with good reason. A whole wheat grain contains over 30 known nutrients and is made up of a few parts: the bran, the middlings, the germ, and the germ oil. Once those are removed, you get what's left: white flour. These are removed because they drastically reduce the shelf-life. But the wheat industry is smart, they're not throwing the rest of the stuff away, they're selling it separately as health food. It's a great way for them to make money, and a very bad way for you to consume flour. What are the options then?

If you are so inclined, you can get a grain mill and make your own flour. The initial cost of a grain mill can be a little pricey, but you will save money in the long run making your own flour as it is much cheaper to purchase wheat, spelt, rye, and other grains in bulk. Left in their original state and properly stored, these dried grains will last a very long time. The health benefits are enormous, though, as you are able to get fresh flour that contains all of its original parts. If you've never smelled fresh flour, it is a beautiful thing. Foodies, if you haven't gone there, you've missing a whole new world.

If you're interested in consuming grains, your options from best to worst (nutritionally) are:

1. Freshly whole milled organic sprouted grains.
2. Organic whole grains or sprouted grains.
3. Whole grains.
4. White fluff flour and the evil concoctions made from it.

Action steps

Because everyone is in a different spot on their food journey, your action steps may look different for the next few weeks. What resonates with you the most? Start there. Do you feel a little voice challenging you to give up dairy for a little while to experiment? If so, I encourage you to try. Are you ready to ditch the sodium nitrates and nitrites and seek out quality meats? Go. Pick one very specific goal (example: over the next two weeks, I will purchase produce on the Dirty Dozen list organically) and make it happen.

There are a lot of different goals that you may have that will filter out through this chapter. If that is the case, write them all down and pick the order that you want to tackle them in. You do not need to do everything all at once. Walk in, eyes open, and pay attention to how your body feels once you adopt a new practice.

Chapter 4: Quasi-Foodlike Substances that Maybe You Shouldn't Eat

Two-week goal: Consider removing a foodlike substance and replace it with real food, or a choice that is more beneficial for you.

Michael Pollan (the author of *The Omnivore's Dilemma*) and others like him have been telling us to "eat real food" for a long time. In fact, his tagline is, "Eat food. Not too much. Mostly plants." I was watching an interview once with him and the interviewer asked him how to eat. His response was something like, "Only eat real food." What does that mean?

It means if it walked on two or four legs, grew from the ground, lived in the ocean, grew on a tree – you can (probably) eat it. If it was made in a lab – don't eat it. If it was processed so far that it doesn't even resemble anything in nature – don't eat it. If it contains an abbreviation – don't eat it. If it was genetically modified – don't eat it.

Prepare to wrap your brain around something phenomenal – that is, the food we eat, every single bite, is information to our cells and programs our genetic expression. According to Dr. David Perlmutter, a neurologist, author, and Fellow at the college of American College for Nutrition, the food you choose to eat changes the expression of your DNA, either fostering a proper cellular life cycle, or promoting an abnormal one. A new field of science is blossoming called nutrigenomics, which focuses on how the molecules in our food interact with our genes to support health. This is no longer the usual plea from the fashion magazine on the grocery store check-out rack appealing to your vanity (although eating properly will most definitely change your body for the better) – yanking your heartstrings with your desire to look smokin' hot in yoga pants or that primal manly, testosterone-laden desire to rid yourself of your beer gut and love handles and return to your GQ model six-pack of old. This is a cry for you to recognize that you are programming your genetic expression and increasing your chance for improved survival with every bite that you put in your mouth.

We are neglecting (to our own detriment!) the notion that food is information. Everything that we put into our body can either nourish and build us up or foster a state of disease, weakness, and stress. Does it not seem to make greater sense that when your body is already in a state of exhaustion for you to feed it properly and give it strength so that you can do what you must? You have so many things that you must accomplish on a daily basis, and people to take care of, but if you are denying yourself the best fuel, you are limiting your chances at success. This is insane. We are perpetuating a downhill spiral of less than optimal health, while expecting ourselves to ignore biology and somehow magically rise to overcome the challenge, with no thought for the toll that it takes on our bodies. We need to wake up. One cannot make something from nothing, nor can we make withdrawals on a physical bank account when there haven't been any worthy deposits made.

One of the other main reasons that so many people find it difficult to eat real food at home is because junk food and fast food are actually physically addictive. Your brain is not imagining it, and it is not merely a matter of having more willpower. As you sit there and contemplate whether to have a nice kale salad or a burger from the fast food place on the corner, that strong desire to have the latter is based also in your biology. The scientists who design fast food do so with the motive that you will want more of it, and will specifically want their brand and what they have created. In *Salt, Sugar, Fat: How the Food Giants Hooked Us* by Michael Moss, we see the very blatant and near sinister workings of an industry that depends on "mouthfeel" and a careful balance between salt, sugar, and fat to find your "blisspoint". This balance between these three powerhouses makes it impossible for your brain to distinguish a weight on any one of them, which would cause you to stop eating and be satiated. You will recognize this when you eat something that is quite salty – you get sick of it after not too long. The same with something that is too sweet or too fatty. But when these three are in a balance that your brain cannot solidly detect one over the other, you spin into an uncontrollable cycle of eating because you are receiving positive feedback from hitting all of those pleasure centers in your brain, while not overpowering any of them. Food scientists know this and use it to their advantage. Think of the delicious tortilla chip – a little salty, sweet from the corn, and fat from the oil – it is a dangerous mix against your willpower. Added to the science are chemicals like monosodium glutamate, a neurotoxic sodium-based amino acid that acts as a flavor enhancer, activating the pleasure centers of your brain. Your brain then ties that specific food and brand to pleasure, which develops a biological craving.

The opposite of this is true. If you ask anyone who has been away from fast food for a while, the palate will change enough to be able to appreciate the nuances and sweetness and unique flavors within real food, making it a pleasure to experience. When someone is offered fast food who has been away from it for a long time, it no longer has the addictive power it once may have had. The solution is to get onto the other side of addiction, and although an uphill climb, it can be done. It's done through eating real food until not only your body realizes that fake food is fake, but your taste buds do, and are repulsed by it.

Sound impossible? It isn't. If it worked for me, "Mountain Dew Girl", it can work for you.

Let me persuade you a little further with one more wonderful benefit of eating real food - you are more easily satiated and less hungry all of the time. When your body is getting nutritional markers checked off, it stops demanding so much of a constant supply of fuel. Our cravings do mean something and it is important to listen to our bodies, but we have a tendency to fill it with the wrong thing so it never gets the signal to shut off. If your body is craving salt, it is likely seeking the spectrum of minerals that quality salt provides (like grey Celtic sea salt). If you feed it white table salt, you'll never fill up what it's looking for, whether that is manganese, magnesium, boron, copper, or other trace minerals your body needs to function because it does not exist in refined table salt. (A note on white table salt – it does contain added iodine, but it also bleached and contains anti-caking agents. If you need iodine, you may be better off looking elsewhere.) This is why it is possible for some people to eat an entire bag of chips: the blisspoint of salt, sugar, and fat combined with the lack of minerals in the salt never give your body the signal to stop. You get to the bottom of the bag and you're still not satiated, and looking for something else. It is a twisted and genius way for the food giants to make money, but your health and vigor are sacrificed on that altar. Stand up for your body and protect it. You're the gatekeeper to what is allowed to infiltrate your castle.

You're not crap, so don't eat crap. You're worth giving your body good things. Give your biology a boost until your brain agrees. Every bite counts. Make it count for your team. This is not a time to sink into leftover mentality. Give appropriately to yourself so you can be effective in this life and pour out for others.

Quick tips for avoiding bad food cravings:
1. Drink more water. Sometimes you think you're hungry but you're dehydrated instead. Start with water.

2. Brush your tongue or use a tongue scraper. Do you ever eat delicious vanilla Joe Joe's one night and want them so bad again the next? Microscopic bits are left behind on your tongue, sending signals up to your brain, telling you to hook it up and fork over the Joe Joe's again. Brush that away and you'll work in parallel with your biology.
3. Say yes to nutrition – veggies, fruits, clean protein – and your body is much more likely to be satiated.
4. Don't make something completely taboo. You're a rebel, we all know it. If you tell yourself you'll never eat a cookie again and that cookies are off the list, you're going to dream about cookies until you have one. You will give it an unreasonable amount of power in your life. Take it off of the unattainable shelf. What if you gave yourself permission? Would you really eat a whole box? Or do you eat a whole box because you're not supposed to?
5. Reward yourself with other wonderful things. McDonald's isn't a reward, it's a punishment. Get a massage, go see a movie, connect with a friend, or do something you've never done before but always wanted to. Those experiences are much more enriching to your life than a double cheeseburger.

Alcohol

Alcohol is obviously not a food, but it is something that is important to mention if we're aiming for your better health. Drinking in moderation is not inherently unhealthy, but very few people have a practical handle on what the definition of "drinking in moderation" really is. Out of all of the categories of food, I can't think of anything that a person would not like to hear more than something along the lines of telling them that they drink too much. I understand that and know it is a delicate subject, but if you have goals that you want to get to and alcohol is something that is standing in your way, or if you are hurting yourself and birthing health issues as a result, as your health coach, I'm going to do the very undesirable and uncomfortable thing and call you to account for it.

"Drinking in moderation" has an actual definition, and is outlined in the U.S. Dietary Guidelines. One drink is equivalent to 5 ounces of wine (12% alcohol), 12 ounces of regular beer (5% alcohol), or 1.5 ounces of

80-proof distilled liquor (40% alcohol). Women are allowed a maximum of one drink per day and a maximum of 7 drinks per week. Men are double that – two drinks per day (although, please, no, just, no) and a maximum of 14 drinks per week.

Go to your kitchen and grab a measuring cup. Notice the marks for 1.5 ounces, 5 ounces, and what 12 ounces would be. Is that less or more than what you would drink?

Heavy drinking is considered drinking more than three drinks in one day for women or exceeding the 7 drinks per week threshold. For men, it's drinking more than four drinks in one day or having more than 14 in a week. Binge drinking is one more step up and includes a shorter time factor. If within two hours, you're female and drink four or more drinks or male and drink five or more, you're bingeing. Neither one of these categories is a good place to be for your health.

I am a proud graduate of Michigan State University and I am fully aware that a lot of people do not drink within the realms of moderation. (In fact, that burning couch belonged to my friend, so I am no stranger to what binge drinking looks like.) Besides the obvious problems with heavy drinking and binge drinking of being considered somewhat of an alcoholic, there are other health considerations that you may want to pay attention to. Excessive alcohol consumption is the third leading cause of premature death in the United States (after smoking and obesity)[8], and as you've just seen, "moderate" alcohol use seems to be closer to what society would deem as "minimal" alcohol use, and "excessive" as what many people consider normal.

1. Cancer and alcohol[9]

The risk of cancer increases significantly with alcohol use. Although researchers do not know the exact function that makes alcohol a carcinogenic substance, it is speculated by the current evidence that it has to do with the metabolism of acetaldehyde, the main metabolite of ethanol; an increase in estrogen concentration (which increases the risk of breast, ovarian, and cervical cancer); that it acts as a solvent for tobacco carcinogens (because, social smoking), it messes with your B vitamins, and causes free radical damage (which ages you and leads to degenerative diseases). Alcohol increases the risk of liver, colon, rectal, pancreatic, and mouth/throat/esophageal cancer. If you have a family history of any of these cancers, or if you exhibit other risk factors for these cancers (not getting enough fiber, eating processed lunchmeats, smoking, using tobacco, etc.), you need to think seriously about the costs and benefits of how much you are drinking.

2. Alcohol and obesity

There aren't a ton of positives for your health in regards to alcohol consumption. If you're really digging, you can pull out that there's resveratrol in red wine, but it balances against the sugar, empty calories, and alcohol that it's providing your body along with it. If one of your goals is to lose weight but you are consistent in drinking copious amounts of alcohol, you're working against yourself. Indeed, binge drinking is associated with a greater risk of obesity and waist circumference.[10] BMI, waist circumference, and waist to hip ratio were significantly increased when men drank 21 drinks or more per week.[11] Another interesting finding with alcohol consumption is that it is also positively related to consuming more food while drinking. Perhaps that is a social construct – we drink with friends, and eat, too. Or perhaps it is a biological response. Because alcohol is empty calories (not a ton of nutrition, fiber, etc.), your body still is going to ask you to fill in those nutritional holes it needs to function for the day, so in many cases you may just end up drinking a bunch more than you would have, and piling on the food too. It doesn't take rocket science to figure out that this is the opposite behavior you want for weight loss.

3. Alcohol and depression

Here is another chicken-egg dilemma. Alcohol use is related to depression. Many people who are depressed seek to find avenues to ameliorate their pain and discomfort, and alcohol is a quick and (mostly) socially acceptable means of doing so. Whether you rely on it to calm you down after a stressful or difficult day, are consuming it to blunt the heart-trauma your life is dealing you, or your drinking has set you into depression, the unfortunate truth is that the research shows that both situations exist: that is, alcohol-induced depression, and depression-induced alcoholism (which women are more susceptible to).[12] I know that this is not a popular belief, nor is it an easy one, but I believe that in order to move through the pain that life deals us, we need to walk into it, through it, and let it hit us. Sometimes it is overwhelmingly emotionally distressing, seemingly unfair, and you experience the physical and debilitating pain of a broken heart, wishing things could be different so often that your mind is clouded and you don't even recognize yourself anymore. I think strength comes from walking through those fires, even though walking looks more like crawling, limping, and being incapacitated on most days, fake smiling your way until you can be alone again to let the pain burn through you. Don't always run away. Don't drown your feelings. Alcohol is not going to help you. It is a fickle friend in those times.

This is not a diatribe for teetotalism, but I wish to present this information to you so that you can make an informed, personal decision regarding what you ought to do in respect to your alcohol consumption. I'm not going to tell you what to do on this, but I am going to inform you so that you know what you're getting into.

What I will tell you is that if you do decide to drink alcohol to give your body a boost beforehand to counteract the negatives. When your body has an influx of alcohol, your liver tries to process it out. Your liver's job is to break alcohol down with an enzyme. Alcohol is broken down into acetaldehyde, but acetaldehyde is thirty times more toxic than alcohol. Your body then tries to break the acetaldehyde down again with a different enzyme into acetate, which is harmless (and similar to vinegar). This is a genius design. The problem occurs when your body runs out of the second enzyme (it's called acetaldehyde dehydrogenase) from too much drinking. (And women naturally have less of it in their bodies than men, which is why it is more common for females to be more severely affected than males by alcohol consumption.) That looks like liver damage, alcohol poisoning, and hangovers.

N-acetyl cysteine (NAC) is an amino acid that helps reduce acetaldehyde toxicity and can be taken before you drink to lessen hangover effects. (At least 200 mg is needed.) B vitamins are also depleted in the body, so taking B1 and B6 before drinking will help (B vitamins also work synergistically and better with NAC). Magnesium and vitamin C are two other supplements that you may benefit from taking before drinking alcohol as vitamin C has protective effects for your liver, and magnesium is anti-inflammatory but depleted with alcohol use.

Please also stay hydrated with water and electrolytes while you're consuming alcohol. Eat food before and while you're drinking. Drink coconut water for electrolytes (warning: some people really hate the taste, but suck it up, buttercup. If you can drink alcohol, you can drink coconut water.). Otherwise, don't drink and drive, and potentially don't drink and text (which has its own issues).

May you be able to make good, healthy food and drink decisions for your future, balancing them properly against sucking the life out of life. When it comes down to it, that's what I want for you. I want you to have the energy and the ability to do what you love to do, what you dream of doing, and what you're meant to do on this earth. The information presented in this chapter is birthed out of a passion for you to be able to make educated decisions and to take charge of the direction your ship is headed. You have beautiful things to give. The world can open up to you with a clear mind, good health, and a solid physical capacity. When you are not hindered by illness, brain fog, lethargy, and apathy, you are able to go after your big dreams and make a difference in this world. I want that for you. I'm on your team. Go get it!

Action steps

If you're addicted to fast food and quasi-foodlike substances, make it a point to add in the good rather than holding the mentality of withholding something from yourself. When you add in drinking proper amounts of water and getting the nutrition you need, it is a lot easier to work with your biology and fight the biological craving of junk. Plan ahead. Carry real food in your vehicle so that you're less tempted when you're famished to pull over and eat something that is going to derail you from your goals. Reward yourself with other things that nourish your body instead of self-sabotage where you're trying to be.

If you have a suspicion that you might drink too much or if people who love you have confronted you in this area, get help. If you are drinking in moderation, consider taking a vitamin B supplement to help offset what will be lacking in your body as a result. If you're pretty sure you're going to have a hangover, you may want to try activated charcoal before you go to bed to help pull those toxins from your body. Take care of yourself. Alcohol can be fun, but it can suck the life out of you before you realize it if you let it. Love your body well so it can do what you want it to later.

Chapter 5: Probiotics

Two-week goal: Experiment with probiotic foods or supplements

What if I told you there was something in your body that was connected to mental health, gut health, your immune system, and even was a marker for your ability to lose weight? It seems strange that there could be one thing that crosses all of those lines. It is true and it is nothing short of remarkable.

That one thing is probiotics.

What are probiotics, anyway? Simply put, probiotics are the good guys who live in your gut. (They also live inside of your mouth, in your lady parts, and on your skin.) They are good bacteria and yeasts that populate your intestines and make up about 60-80% of your immune system. They supply essential nutrients, synthesize vitamin K, develop blood vessels, and promote enteric nerve function (the "gut's brain").

Probiotics are relatively new kids on the block in regards to medical research and their function within our bodies, but with each new discovery comes a new level of wonder and appreciation for our unique and wonderful biological system. We have recently found that our bodies contain more microbes than human cells, and not by a little bit. The microbes living in our bodies are near ten times the amount of our human cells.[13] (You're a wonderful host, by the way.) Our guts contain between 500 to 2000 different species of microorganisms – from yeasts, to parasites, to viruses, to bacteria, and more. When things are in balance (which looks like 85% good guys and 15% bad guys), you have a good shot at overall health. When things are out of balance, a whole host (ha!) of things can go wrong.

> **Good sources of prebiotics**
> raw chicory root
> raw garlic
> raw jicama
> under ripe bananas
> raw leeks
> raw asparagus
> raw dandelion greens
> raw or cooked onions
> acacia gum

Our gut is a microbiome with a unique ecosystem. Things can become unbalanced when certain lifestyle or dietary changes are made, including the use of antibiotics, an increase in stress, eating poorly, illness, and aging. Sugar is fuel for the bad guys; whereas certain helpful prebiotics (specific non-digestible fibers) feeds the good guys and increases their proliferation. Stress causes an increase in inflammation in our bodies and has an effect on every cell in our body, gut included. Antibiotics, while an amazing discovery and has saved many lives, are something like the gut equivalent of a nuclear bomb.

The bulk of our immune system is housed in our gut. The genius design of our gut contains a layer only one cell thick, called the endothelium, allowing for easy communication across the barrier regarding the information that is coming in and what our body needs to do with it, but being so thin, it is easy to damage and should be carefully guarded. It is also the location of the bulk of your immune system: the army, navy, and marines of your body.

The incredible design of our body is such that we have two lines of defense – a mechanical barrier and an immune barrier. The mechanical barrier is the single layer of cells (think: building a wall at the border to keep out invaders – insert political comments here), and the immune barrier is the fighter cells. When something bad tries to get in, certain cells will scooch over to the mucosal surface of the colon and take up all of the nutrients and attachment sites so the bad guys have nowhere to go (it's also called "colonization resistance"). It's pushing the bad guys out of the way, taking up all of the room so they can't hang out, and starving them on a microscopic level. The other plan of attack includes shooting up the bad guys with a toxic substance that will stop their growth or kill them. When there is a break in the wall (sometimes referred to as "leaky gut" or intestinal permeability), waste and bad guys that were supposed to be on their way out are able to break on through to the other side, getting in where they ought not be, and wreaking havoc in every direction. Taking care of our intestinal endothelial layer, the good guys, and the fight is of utmost importance. Without them, our line of defense is nothing and we are open to attack from everything that the world is throwing our way.

With this in mind, are you surprised that more than forty diseases have been linked to bacterial imbalances? The more obvious ones are inherently connected to your gut and digestive tract like IBS, Crohn's disease, and ulcerative colitis, but research is now linking gut dysbiosis (the imbalance between the good guys and the bad ones) with obesity, diabetes (type 1 and type 2), NASH (non-alcoholic steatohepatitis), cardiovascular disease, colon and prostate cancer, HIV, AIDS, and autism spectrum disorders.

How do you know if you have an imbalance in your gut bacteria composition? Imbalance is linked to intestinal symptoms as well as other diseases: bloating, abdominal pain, diarrhea, inflammatory bowel disease, obesity, diabetes, liver diseases, chronic heart diseases, cancers, HIV, and autism. An imbalance has also been implicated in bipolar disorder.[14] The microbiome-gut-brain axis is being explored with incredible connections that are certain to change and shape the future of mental health.

If you suffer from any of those problems, is it all lost? Are you doomed to succumb to the host of diseases because of your destroyed endothelial layer or your imbalanced microbiome?

Not if I have anything to say about it.

As you can ascertain, it seems that nearly all of your health is balancing somehow on this critical issue, and certainly a bulk of it is. When you are out of balance, you do not feel well. Your stomach is not happy. You may feel foggy in your brain. You may even be depressed or suffering from cancer or chronic heart disease. This is not the easiest way for you to try to reach your fullest potential. I want you to wake up feeling energized and happy, ready to tackle the world. Let's knock this barrier back and help your body build a good, strong wall, and a happy, well-functioning and properly fed army.

You can do this at least one of two ways.

The first is by taking a probiotic supplement. If you had to go through the unfortunate experience of the nuclear option of your intestines via antibiotics, I would highly recommend that you take this option for a few months to help repopulate your guts with good guys. If you've ever gone to the store in an attempt to purchase some probiotic supplements, you will be amazed at the variety (and the price range). In my opinion, it seems more logical to buy something that actually works than for you to save a little bit of money on something that is completely worthless. You may as well not have spent any money at all in that case.

Probiotic supplements are measured in CFUs. Those are "colony forming units", the approximation of the viable amount of yeast or bacteria in a product. If you nuked your guts, I don't recommend anything less than 50 billion CFUs, and would rather you aim more toward 85 billion CFUs. In general, the refrigerated probiotics usually have a reputation for being more viable than those designated for shelf-stable usage. The controlled temperature allows for a bit more stability, with hopes that more of the good guys will make it alive to you.

Probiotics are amazingly specific. There are versions of probiotics that are formulated for issues more prevalent in men and others designed for women's health. Depending on your specific issues and needs, you will need different strains. The following chart will give you some ideas regarding the support each strain can give you.

L. acidophilus	Overall digestion, absorption of nutrients, relief from gastrointestinal discomforts, immune system health, urinary and vaginal health
L. fermentum	Overall digestion, detoxification
L. plantarum	Overall digestion, immune health
L. rhamnosus	Vaginal health, traveler's diarrhea
L. salivarius	Immune health, oral health
L. paracasei	Liver health
L. gasseri	Vaginal health, relief from occasional diarrhea
L. reuteri	Oral health, immune health, overall digestion
B. bifidum	Overall digestion, nutrient absorption, relief from traveler's diarrhea
B. longum	Overall digestion, detoxification, immune health
B. infantis	Overall digestion, relief from occasional bloating and constipation
B. coagulans	Overall digestion, relief from occasional constipation, vaginal health
S. salivarius K12	Overall oral health, immune health
S. salivarius M18	Healthy teeth and gums

The other means to enhance your microbiome is by consuming foods that support gut health. Traditional diets from all over the world incorporated cultured or fermented foods into almost every meal, and now we can understand the wisdom for doing so. Not only are they easier to digest because the enzymes present have already begun "predigestion", but they also contain a myriad of probiotics. Fermented foods may also be considered the first convenience foods – most fermented foods are soaked or allowed to work over a period of time where cooking was not included (think of kombucha, kimchi, sauerkraut, etc.). After a long day of working, the crock of sauerkraut or raw cheese or beet kvass stood ready for consumption.

Fermented vegetables	sauerkraut kimchi pickles
Fermented grains	sourdough bread kvass kiesiel kisra koji injera
Fermented beans	miso natto tempeh dosa
Fermented dairy	filmjölk cultured butter crème fraiche lassi skyr viili yogurt
Fermented drinks	kombucha şalgam water kefir beet kvass ginger beer

This extremely high tech chart is just a sample of some of the different kinds of cultured and fermented foods across the world.

Some studies showed that the probiotic volume in a serving of cultured foods surpassed an entire bottle's worth of probiotic supplements. Are your ready to dive in?

You may recognize some of the foods in the chart – sourdough bread, yogurt, maybe crème fraiche. I want to point out that (just like everything else) not all yogurts/sauerkrauts/pickles are created equally. If you are planning on increasing your probiotic load through yogurt, take care that you are not choosing a variety that is going to be excessive in sugar or strange and unnecessary ingredients. Fermented pickles and sauerkrauts are made from a brine, and you should not see vinegar or preservatives listed on the ingredient label. And if you're buying sourdough bread, avoid purchasing those with a long list of funky ingredients.

Here are a few (more) common fermented foods that you can find to incorporate into your daily regimen:

1. Yogurt

Look for yogurt sourced from grass-fed whole milk. A teaspoon of sugar is the equivalent of 4 grams. Before you buy your yogurt (or anything else), flip to the back, read the amount of sugar it has in grams, divide it by 4. Picture scooping that amount of sugar from your spoon into the container. If it seems excessive, you may want to make a different choice. We're here to support gut health, not to fuel the bad guys. If you cannot find grass-fed whole milk, choose organic whole milk. I recommend this because cows raised conventionally are usually injected with antibiotics (think: nuclear option) and artificial growth hormones (rBST – think: messing with your endocrine system) and those are passed on to you – neither of which are beneficial for your overall health and wellness.

2. Pickles

Probiotic or cultured pickled vegetables are not the kind you're going to find in the middle of the grocery store sitting on the shelf saturated in vinegar and loaded with strange sodiums. Look for lacto-fermented pickles. If you're adventurous and of a capable nature, you can try your hand at making your own pickled vegetables. Most recipes start with a salt solution brine, some spices, and your vegetables - plus time. The result? Satisfaction for doing things yourself, a high content of probiotics, and a running science experiment in your own space (the mark of cool people everywhere).

3.   Kombucha

Kombucha is a slightly carbonated drink reminiscent of something like a cross between black tea, apple cider vinegar, and beer. Its origin is repudiated to be from Asia – Manchuria, then Japan, and then Russia. The word kombucha means "tea mushroom" (enticing, isn't it?) because it is made by growing a culture in black or green tea. The culture is referred to as a "SCOBY", an acronym meaning "symbiotic culture of bacteria and yeast" which looks like a slippery light colored pancake. Kombucha has become increasingly popular over the last several years as people are beginning to realize the importance of increasing their probiotic load, and as a result, there are quite a few commercial brewers of kombucha. Many offer original or flavored kombucha (for those who can't take it straight). It is also just as easy to brew your own, with significant savings and the ability to tweak your own level of tartness or sweetness. You can have your own batch done between 5 and 15 days, depending on the temperature, and lucky for you, scobies have babies and you can proliferate your supply exponentially.

Kombucha contains something called glucuronic acid. Glucuronic acid is formed in the liver – a substance designed to detoxify the body. It combines with toxins, drugs, and hormones, and transports them out of the body via urine. For people who regularly consume alcohol or certain prescription drugs, the body's ability to produce glucuronic acid is thwarted, which really ends up being a double problem. You need to flush the body of alcohol and excess meds, but the consumption of those inhibits your ability to do so.

If you have ever read the near miracle working properties of kombucha, the "elixir of immortality", you will be shocked and surprised. Fantastic claims that kombucha has cured grey hair, cancer, AIDS, liver disease, joint pain, and a host of other issues are pervasive. I would suggest that kombucha is not a cure, rather, it is something that aids the body in functioning at a more optimal level by supporting liver detoxification and introducing a host of good probiotics to the gut. If your liver is happy and can clean you out, your whole body will benefit. Being that many diseases are a result of inflammation, toxicity, and infection, it is no wonder that something that is able to support detoxification (through the introduction of glucuronic acid), reduce inflammation (through the introduction of probiotics), and infection (also through probiotics – by sending in more good troops) has been linked to such claims.

4. Sauerkraut

Sauerkraut is fermented cabbage. As with pickles, the ingredients to your sauerkraut should just be the vegetable (in this case, cabbage), salt, and water. If you've flipped the bottle around and see anything else, just no. Skip that brand and go for something else. Or, better yet, make sauerkraut at home. Sauerkraut is an amazing food. Cabbage is high in vitamin K, Vitamin C, dietary fiber, folate, B6 and manganese. When it is fermented, the process opens up the cell walls and allows for a higher ratio of vitamins.

Dr. Mercola had a team test the probiotic content in a few ounces of sauerkraut to find just how many colony forming units were present. In 4-6 ounces of sauerkraut (one serving), they found ten trillion CFUs. Some of the very highest probiotic supplements sold today have 85 billion CFUs – that's like taking 117 servings of a very good probiotic supplement in just a few ounces of sauerkraut. Even if you've never tried sauerkraut or hate it, perhaps armed with this information you could find it in your heart to at least take it medicinally.

There are a few brands that make a few varieties of sauerkraut, but my favorite by far is by a thriving company, The Brinery. If you can get your hands on a bottle of their kraut, you'll be impressed. Their product, Sea Stag, contains a whole pile of amazing ingredients, including cabbage, carrots, burdock, turmeric, and sea vegetables. I did not grow up eating such things, so initially it was a challenge. If you happen to fall into that category too, let me encourage you to keep at it. Just like anything else, where there's a will, there's a way. It's an amazing addition to your guts and you're worth it.

5. Water kefir

Water kefir is made from little clear-ish "grains" that eat up and ferment sugar water. The word "kefir" comes from a Turkish word "keif", which means "good feeling". They are reported to originate either in Mexico (with documentation in the late 1800s) or in Tibet, the Caucasus Mountains, and the Ukraine and are thought to have been around for centuries. They are also a symbiotic culture of good bacteria and yeast (like the SCOBY of kombucha). Water kefir is a great choice for those who are allergic, intolerant, or avoiding dairy, as well as those who must avoid caffeine.

Water kefir "grains" can be ordered online or purchased in some health food stores. When they are purchased, they are usually sold dried and you rehydrate them with sugar water. The turnaround time for batching kefir is much shorter than kombucha – between 24-48 hours. Water kefir by itself is not very remarkable, but when double fermented in a fruit juice, it makes for an amazing sweet and fizzy drink. I often double ferment with organic tart cherry juice because of the anti-inflammatory properties.

One warning on water kefir – if you choose to make your own, it is important to regularly burp your bottles in the double fermentation process. Ask me how I know I found out.

One more note, water kefir grains cannot be used to ferment milk. The cultures are different and not interchangeable.

6. Milk kefir

Milk kefir is made from small white grains that eat up and ferment milk. It is similar to a drinkable yogurt for consistency and taste. The origins are unclear, but some say that it was brought over to Chile from migrants of the former Ottoman Empire. For people who are lactose intolerant, milk kefir seems to lack the unpleasant side effects that consumption of regular pasteurized milk brings about. Milk kefir can be made with cow, goat, or sheep's milk, and even milk substitutes like almond and rice.

The benefits of milk kefir are wonderful and surprising. Some studies have pointed that regular consumption of milk kefir has stopped the growth of tumors in mice, especially in breast cancer. The lactic acid present in milk kefir allows it to detoxify by binding itself to and killing aflatoxins and funguses. It has also been reported to build bone density, cure IBS and IBD, prevents asthma, and improves lactose intolerance.

Your mental health link

The fantastic and complex brain-microbiome-gut axis is one of the newer frontiers in biology, and although researchers have been aware that our microbiome influences our central nervous system for some time, the depth of impact and the vast nature in which it does so is astonishing. There is bidirectional communication between your gut and your brain. Isn't that amazing? Think about that - your gut communicates with your brain!

The way that researchers are testing the influence of the microbiome on the central nervous system and the brain is by observing germ-free animals and the effects on their mental health. A germ-free animal is essentially an animal with an absent microbiome. Their gut is void of the trillions of probiotic organisms, and thus, researchers are able to see what effects that has on brain function. What they have found is very interesting - an imbalance of the good bacteria contributes to a risk of disease by increasing low-grade chronic systemic inflammation, increased stress reactivity, increased anxiety, and increased depressive behaviors. These markers all infer that mental health is linked to and influenced by the happy probiotics living in your gut.

This has led to the advent of psychobiotics – live organisms, which, when taken in sufficient amounts, are used to treat psychiatric illnesses. The use of psychobiotics is not just for anxiety disorders or clinical depression – it has been found to have a positive influence on and to be supportive of those experiencing low mood, chronic stress, and symptoms of anxiety. I may be going out on a limb here, but I would have to say that that is the majority of the first world populations.

How is this possible? Our gut produces serotonin, GABA (gamma amino-butyric acid), acetylcholine, and catecholamines. Those neurotransmitters signal brain function and affect behavior. The good guys in the gut also help regulate and control inflammation. When your body is in a state of chronic inflammation, your immune system is turned on and on overdrive. Chronic inflammation in the body looks like a lot of diseases (every "-itis" in the book) and is a signal that your body is really ticked off at you. Chronic inflammation in the brain is known to be the main underlying cause of depression (and other mood and cognitive disorders). There is also a connection between the HPA (hypothalamic-pituitary-adrenal) axis, which is your body's stress response system. When things are out of whack, you are going to feel like a stressball and not be able to manage what is flying at you.

Probiotics (and psychobiotics) have been shown to help lower stress levels. An interesting study was done with stressed out medical school students. Eight weeks before a significant exam, one group was made to drink a probiotic milk kefir drink while the control group drank a placebo milk drink. They drank it every day leading up to the exam. They tested their serotonin, cortisol, and plasma L-tryptophan levels at different points throughout and found that the group drinking the probiotic drink had significantly lower levels of stress. Interestingly enough, they tested their levels two weeks after the exam and found the milk kefir group had significantly higher levels of serotonin and noticed that the control group had an increased rate in abdominal and cold symptoms. (This isn't surprising because we know that the bulk of our immune system is housed in our gut and revolves around a balance of good bacteria. We also know that the presence of good bacteria also helps reduce inflammation, which can cause pain – abdominally or otherwise.)

What does this mean for you? Are you stressed out? Do you suffer from mild or clinical depression? Do you deal with anxiety? Experimenting with a probiotic supplement or introducing probiotic foods and drinks into your daily regimen could help reduce these symptoms and help you feel better and happier.

Some interesting studies

If you're not into being healthy for the sake of being healthy and living with a higher quality of life for longer, I will now appeal to your vanity. (You're welcome. Hey, it is my goal to reach everyone.) Scientists were wondering if and how probiotics and obesity were related to one another, so they did an experiment on mice to find out. They fed mice a diet that included probiotics (lactobacillus gasseri) and took metrics for body weight, fat tissue mass, liver fat content and inflammatory genes in the adipose (fatty) tissue, and lipogenic and lipolytic genes in the liver. What happened? They noticed a significant level of weight loss and fat tissue, as well as a reduction of the triglyceride count in the liver![15] They did not exercise more. They did not change their overall diet. They simply added probiotics to their diet and found these results. Perhaps the presence of more bacteria made it possible for the mice to get nutrients out of what they were eating, making the body function better. Perhaps the presence of more good guys reduced inflammation, which promoted obesity. Perhaps it was something else entirely, but the encouraging results speak for themselves.

Other studies in humans have shown similarly interesting and shocking results. Researchers wanted to get down and dirty studying the different microbiomes of obese and lean people. How did they do this? You'll be so glad you wondered: fecal cultures. The researchers consistently found that obese people had less variety and fewer numbers of beneficial bacteria and yeasts in their gut than their leaner counterparts. Are you ready for the next horizon in the science of weight loss and obesity? (You're not, I can assure you.) Poop transfers. Technically, it's called fecal microbiome transplantation, but even that word is going out of vogue (can you imagine?) because of the near inherent association with the unhygienic and dirty. The new (cleaner) terminology is "gut microbiome transplantation" (GMT), and I'm sure you can imagine why. Scientists have taken some (ahem) gut microbiota from lean people and transferred it to obese people. The results have all been positive, increasing insulin sensitivity by 75%, and a better gut outcome of more species and a higher population of the helpful bacteria. The reverse has also proven true – that is, when a lean person was inoculated with the gut microbiota of an obese person, they gained weight. (This study was done originally to test for different cures of repeated *C. difficile* infections.)

So it's like this: Are you unhappy with your current weight and amount of body fat? Do you want to be more lean? Bump up your probiotics. (Or seek to be one of the first on your block to get a gut microbiome transplantation…)

Action Steps

Over the next two weeks, I want to encourage you to speak with your doctor and seek out different sources of probiotics and try them to see what works best for you. Some people are highly sensitive to probiotics, depending on their biological makeup and current state of their microbiome. If you experience diarrhea or other digestive issues as a result of taking them, you may need to slow down your intake and slowly build up. As an example, when people first try kombucha for the first time, I suggest that they try about 4 ounces a day for a week to see how they feel. If all is well, the next week they bump to 6 ounces. The following week moves up to 8 ounces, and after that, whatever their body is craving.

As with any new regimen, you should speak with your doctor to make sure it is right for you.

Chapter 6:
Exercise: Pump It Up

Two-week goal: Introduce movement that you love into your routine

I squinted up at the light, walking briskly while watching the snow streaming down in white contrast against the black pre-dawn sky. I pulled my parka tighter around me, the subzero temps made worse by the gusts of icy wind. Being a creature of habit, I was motivated to hurry in to get my locker because they'd be here today. It was a little after 5:00 a.m. on January 2, and the Resolutionists would be arriving to mingle for the next three to four weeks. I've always held curiosity for the phenomenon, no matter where I fell in relation to it.

Resolutionists? Yes. Oh, you know. You've probably been one a few times (I have). Perhaps this is an American construct, so for those of you not quite familiar, I'll share with you how a Resolutionist is born.

It begins sometime in October when Halloween candy goes on sale. People begin to pick up a bag or two here or there, convincing themselves that they'll just stock up on candy for the trick-or-treaters, and plus it's on sale, so let's just be festive and buy another orange and black bag (buy two, get one free, yes, please). After a short time, you've got all the Halloween candy you can stand, and you're fully addicted to sugar skipping into November.

November hits and it's Thanksgivemas, the official season of eating to exhaustion in these United States. (This is a sport that we can all get into.) We're already totally addicted to sugar from the Halloween madness but it's time to step into something a little more hearty – excess turkey, gallons of potatoes, and piles of pies. (Can you just put some marshmallows on top of the sweet potatoes? Great, thanks.) The leaders of the pack have stretched their stomachs to impressive levels, and not even a large meal can satisfy. You've got to supersize everything to really even feel it.

But we're not finished yet, because hitting that last turn throws us into holiday parties like Christmas and Hanukkah, with the amount of eating becoming something like the final four championship extreme edition, and you're eating entire giant meals thrice a day, or participating in something akin to an eating marathon that lasts all day long. Gone are the days and thoughts of restraint because this, my dear, is a holiday. And holidays are special and we only do it once a year and it's *all in moderation* anyway.

So we imbibe and gluttonize, waving the magic moderation wand over the top of every meal and hit the last day of the year. Now it's time to drink. And drink some more. And then just a few more, because why would we stop? Until you forget all of your problems of the past year and make grand new ones for yourself for the upcoming one.

Then you wake up on New Year's Day, hung over, unshaven, wearing the most awful red and green plaid pajamas and some weird bunny slippers you got as a white elephant gift, staring repulsed at yourself in the mirror. You feel like you've been run over by a truck and the new pants you got for Christmas don't even fit you because you've gained fifteen pounds since the day before Thanksgiving and now all of your Black Friday shopping deals were for nothing.

That's when you feel the utter disgust and you take inventory. You stand in front of that mirror, sloppy and hideous and lumpy and say the words you've said before, but this time you mean it. You *really* mean it. "That's *it*! I'm going to change. I can't stand it anymore! I feel like a fat, lumpy, greasy, gross-o. I'm going to eat right and work out! That's it! I'll start tomorrow!"

You dig out the exercise pants from the bottom of your drawer (thank goodness they're stretchy and you bought them last year at the same time so they'll fit exactly right), throw them in your gym bag with your running shoes and your gym pass and set your alarm for the crack of dawn.

And then you hit the gym and take my locker.

I am passionate about exercise and movement now (swimming being so near and dear to my heart), but I haven't always been so consistent. It seems like exercise can fall into the classic transtheoretical model quite easily: people recognizing there may be a problem (that is, they want to be stronger, or lose weight, or be faster, or impress that cute girl), wanting to do something about it (maybe work out for a little while) until they self-sabotage and convince themselves that they were right (I exercised for ten minutes four days in a row, why am I still in the same pants size?), they just aren't cut out for movement and exercise (see, I knew it wouldn't work!), it isn't pleasant (everything hurts and I'm dying), and even though they ought to do it, they don't want to (forget it, pass the chips and beer).

This is exactly the problem. Exercise is seen as a chore, as something that is taking away from you. I think what we must start to do is move from a place of "have to" to a place of "want to". But before you can get there, you have to know what you want to do, what you like to do. Your self-determination can take you a long way, but when you love something, you look forward to doing it. But how on earth do you get yourself to like doing something and convince yourself you want to do it when you just don't?

One way for you to raise your level of enjoyment and accountability for movement and exercise is to connect with a friend or two, sign up for a personal training session (or a series), enroll in a class, or join a club. I have to admit something that you may find strange. I love waking up before 5:00 in the morning to go swimming. I leap out of bed, excited to do it. Why? I swim with around 20 determined, driven, and intelligent people on a Master's swim team long before the sun comes up and I know that if I don't show up for a week (let's be honest - a few days, I'm addicted), they are going to wonder where I am. There is camaraderie within the normalcy of our insanity. Face it, when you wake up that early to jump in a cold pool to push your body hard for an hour, your life is obviously not characterized by being average (I've heard people throw around the word "crazy" a few times, but I digress). At one time it was hard, but now it is fun, and something I look forward to four or five days a week. The physical release, the delicious chlorine scent, and the full-body workout is my favorite way to start a day. I've already accomplished something wonderful by 6:30 a.m. – and productivity begets more, and drives you forward to obliterate the list that lurked in front of you upon waking up.

The added accountability of a class or a team will give you an extra layer of willpower and enjoyment because you are able to incorporate a little social time and connection into your workout. By joining a class, you are inherently participating in something with a group of people who have a common interest, and so are a little bit like you right off the bat. Instant camaraderie through shared awesomeness.

Now think through for a moment and consider what you enjoy. One of the things I like to speak with my clients about is the type of exercise or movement that may resonate with them. People's personalities seem to tie in with the sort of exercise they like. Maybe you haven't exercised or done a lot of movement in a very long time and you really don't know what you like, or nothing sounds interesting. Can I encourage you to think back to your childhood to things that you used to like to do?

Did you enjoy riding your bike? Climbing trees? Dance? Gymnastics? Running and playing tag? Walking along rivers, exploring? Maybe you played baseball or hockey or swam. These things are all available to you today! If there is not a local club or class, I encourage you to be the founder of it and get others to participate. Why not? It is likely that others have an interest and are looking for an outlet. Exercise does not have to look like you waking up and lifting weights for an hour before you eat breakfast (although it most certainly can if you're into that).

Blood Type	Japanese Blood Type Personality Chart	Potential Exercise and Movement Interests
A	Sensible, reserved, patient, good listeners, detail oriented, analytical, creative, inventive, responsible, cautious, stubborn, tense, obsessive, pessimistic	Yoga, tai chi, meditation, walking, deep breathing
B	Passionate, active, creative, flexible, cheerful, optimistic, irresponsible, forgetful, lazy, selfish, unreliable	Tennis, martial arts, biking, golf, hiking
AB	Cool, controlled, adaptable, rational, intelligent, indecisive, critical, indecisive, unforgiving, aloof	Alternating intense exercise with very calming exercises: i.e., three days of aerobic exercise like running or biking followed by two days of yoga or tai chi
O	Confident, self-determined, ambitious, strong-willed, intuitive, agreeable, competitive, athletic, self-centered, cold, aggressive, unpredictable, arrogant, ruthless	Aerobic activity like swimming, running, biking, hiking, kickboxing, cross country skiing

There is a thought-provoking belief out there that connects your blood type to your personality and your preferred type of movement and exercise. I want to share these with you because it may be helpful for you to connect to different ideas that you may not have had before to help you stir things up and make them interesting. These may or may not resonate with you, but it may give you something to think about.

Think of the things you loved to do as you were growing up and reconnect with them. This is a key in finding the desire to exercise, even when you hate exercising. Does it count as exercise if you are doing something you love, something that is fun? Of course it does. Don't be stuck in the construct that exercise has to be horrible torture. Instead, it can be torturously awesome. Remember those things that you love. Movement is many things and it does not serve you to think the only exercise that counts is running and lifting weights. If you hate those things, what is the point? Walk and listen to a podcast, go kayaking, sign up for a dance class with your bestie. Connect yourself with what you love and with what you think is fun. There are so many possibilities out there, and some will fit you just right.

Sometimes it is inspiring to imagine yourself working to become a certain type of athlete. Wouldn't it be cool to be a marathon runner (or even just a runner in general)? What about picturing yourself as a triathlete? Or the fastest female in your age group in the state for the 400 IM (which, incidentally, is probably easy because nobody in their right mind swims that anyway)? These are not unattainable. Every athlete starts somewhere. If you can make small steps toward reaching those goals, you can become anything you dream up.

When I was in high school and college, I participated in sports and in club activities, but once I graduated and got married, there were not a lot of opportunities for group sports (besides church softball teams and my dodge ball birthday parties, of course). I wasn't a runner, but I thought that I would like to become one (it seemed like a quality I should have), so I told my then high school cross country team member sister that I would like to run a marathon. She looked at me, slightly bewildered and surprised, and gently asked me if I knew what a marathon was. Nope, I sure didn't. After she informed me that it was a 26.2-mile race, I no longer thought that was a very good idea and asked her what other kinds of races were available. She cut distance in half and in half again until she hit the magic number: a 5k.

I signed myself up for one. I had never been able to run more than a block without being so winded that I had to stop and check if my lungs were bleeding, but the desire I had to be able to call myself a runner made me push forward. I ran every day in preparation for my race. A competitive nature did not allow me to do anything other than practice and I found my motivation: I imagined the females in my age group out there every day, hitting the pavement, digging deep, running faster and farther. I imagined what I would have to do to beat them. And then I imagined myself passing the men. It worked for me and I began to love it.

I completed my first 5k a couple months after I had a baby. It was so rewarding and worthwhile, I was immediately hooked. I find this resonates especially well with stay-at-home parents. Quite honestly, there isn't a lot of positive feedback and cheering for you while you load the wet clothes into the dryer, scrub the floors, prepare the dinner, wash the dishes, and clean globs of toothpaste out of the sink. You don't get a thank you note for sitting up with your baby when she's crying and coughing with croup, and you don't get a sorry when your little guy throws up all over you. But do you know what happens when you do a 5k? People stand on the sides of the streets and clap and scream for you. Sometimes they hold up signs and tell you you're kicking butt. There's a finish line waiting for you, telling you that you really accomplished something (unlike the perpetual pile of dishes that magically appears on the scene of your daily life, mocking your work with their "I'm baaaack" attitudes).

Sometimes you even *get a medal*!

(I must warn you: you may get addicted. This was a gateway drug for me. It started with 5ks, and then I did a 10k. Next thing you know, I was training for a half-marathon and getting into triathlons. Once you hit those, the sky is the limit and you're dreaming of Boston and Kona, and a good time on a Saturday morning in the summer entails you swimming miles in local ponds with a bunch of other crazy addicts who do ultramarathons and 10k open water swims for fun.)

Besides finding a group of people or a team to enjoy movement with, one other way to avoid boredom within your exercise routine is to mix it up. Cross training is not only great for helping push you further in your primary exercise, but the change gives you something to look forward to.

You can even alter the types of exercise within a certain category to keep things fresh – choose a day for sprints, longer distance, lower body, circuits, upper body, technique work, or even finding a different location to do your workouts.

When I am training for a triathlon, changing up exercise is easy as it is built in to the very nature of the sport. You may swim several days a week, but you must also incorporate running and biking. I change my running and biking locations and distances so I do not get bored of the same scenery, and then on other days I will lift weights or play team sports (like volleyball) or hike. Interestingly enough, this has done more for my speed (specifically in running) than training by only running five days a week. I ran my best 5k time on the end of a sprint triathlon, and it is due to the amount of cross training that is inherent to multisport. Keep things interesting for yourself and make a plan to do various activities – this will keep you more motivated, more interested, and even more physically fit overall.

Do you need the cold hard facts as to why your body wants you to do this? I want to share with you some very interesting research about physical exercise and how it relates to the rest of your body and overall health.

Good reason #1: It makes your brain work better and helps you to avoid degenerative diseases like Alzheimer's and dementia[16]

Alzheimer's and dementia are on the rise. Assisted living homes are filled with the shells of once vibrant, active, intelligent people who now are shadows of who they once were. They are drugged, laying in beds, kicking backward in their wheelchairs down the halls yelling incomprehensible things, and unable to care for their own basic needs. This is not how it has to be.

If you are to avoid this fate in your advanced age, you need to take steps now to avoid it. Among other things like fueling your brain with omega 3 fish oil, getting enough healthy fats, and avoiding aluminum exposure (via canned foods, Brita/Pur/Culligan water pitchers, baked goods on aluminum trays, vaccination adjuvants, and aluminum foil), you need to engage your body in fighting degenerative disease by exercise. One year of aerobic exercise for seniors increased their hippocampal volumes significantly, and also contributed to better spatial memory and higher cognitive scores.[17]

Essentially, if you want to have a strong brain, you also need to work your body. Everything is connected. Imagine that.

Good reason #2: Aerobic exercise reduces anxiety and depression

If a quarter of your friends aren't on anti-anxiety or antidepressants (SSRIs like Zoloft or Prozac), then you either haven't asked them or they're not telling you the truth. This is reaching a near epidemic level. Nearly 75% of my clients have reported being depressed or anxious – and for some, it interferes with everyday life on a consistent basis. The quick answer from the western medical community is to prescribe such SSRIs (selective serotonin reuptake inhibitors) and to hope for the best. While there are certainly cases where patients need such intervention, many more prescriptions are given out flippantly and easily without many other recommendations.

If you have experienced bouts of depression or anxiety, there is great news for you. Research proves that exercise can kick a lot of it to the curb. Exercise reduces negative mood and increases self-esteem.[18] It increases the blood flow to your brain. Researchers have done studies with a population of the clinically depressed, prescribing exercise for one group, a social support group for another, and a control group (who were told they were on a waiting list).[19] The exercise that was prescribed was walking 20-40 minutes three times a week for six weeks. The authors found that the exercise group had alleviated overall depressive symptoms. Other studies found that people simply walking on a treadmill for 30 minutes for 10 consecutive days produced a clinically relevant and statistically significant result in the reduction of symptoms of depression. This is amazing!

Yes, it is difficult to begin such a thing, especially while depressed, but the rewards that are forthcoming (and so quickly!) may inspire you toward movement. This is great news as it requires no (to a very minimal) investment to get out and walk. Imagine yourself reducing symptoms of depression in only ten days! Do this for yourself. You can do this.

Good reason #3: Exercise reduces high blood pressure, helps prevent heart disease, and stroke

You read that your emotional heart will be happier with exercise, but now your physical heart will be leaping for joy at what you're doing for it. As you exercise that cardiac muscle, you're improving its capabilities to pump your blood throughout your circulatory system, clear waste, battle germs, and carry oxygen and nutrients to your whole body. Your red blood cells and blood vessels grow in size and number as you exercise. Your lungs and heart will function better and be stronger as you incorporate regular physical exercise into your lifestyle and routine. In order for you to get a medicinal level value, you need to engage in aerobic exercise for 30 minutes three times a week.

Good reason #4: You'll have a better sex life

Oh good, I've got your attention now and you're wondering why I didn't list this as reason #1. Listen, it only makes sense. If you're exercising and doing something good for your body, it improves your self-confidence. For men and women, this boosts your happy feelings and makes you more secure and to want to connect intimately with your partner. Improved cardiovascular function and blood flow is vital for men to avoid erectile dysfunction, and with your heart and lungs stronger, you'll be able to run past your sprint straight into a marathon (ahem).

Your heightened physical fitness will help you to feel much better about your body overall, your confidence, your mood, and the most fabulous exercise of all.

Good reason #5: Your creativity will soar[20]

Researchers found that regular exercise improved convergent and divergent thinking, the components for creativity: one is responsible for thinking of one solution to a problem, and the other is responsible for creating multiple solutions. Are you looking for a way to solve that problem that has been bothering you for a while? Employ exercise to loosen what is stuck in your mind, freeing your creativity, and potentially linking you to answers you have been waiting for.

Good reason #6: You will remember things that you learned better

A study was done that showed that people retained more information four hours after they exercised. Do you want to be awesome, strong, and a genius? Look no further. Exercise in the morning, and read a book later. Your brain will suck it up like a sponge and you'll remember what you're studying and learning. (Think of all the possibilities! Foreign language, linear algebra, the history of the English monarchs and their genealogies, memorization of poetry and Shakespearean theater, the intricacies of metamorphic rocks and the water cycle, the list is endless.)

Action steps

1. Write down three of your top options for exercise or movement that you love or that resonates with you.
2. If you are going to participate in a team sport or with other people, contact them and set up a time this week to start. (I'm not kidding. Do it. Like right now. You want to procrastinate, but that is self-sabotage. Tell yourself who is boss, and to suck it up, buttercup.)
3. Tell other people that you are going to begin an exercise routine. Accountability is key. Ask them to ask you about it and how it is going.
4. Do some form of movement and exercise at least three times this week and next.
5. Write down what you've accomplished or track your progress on an app. Write down how long you exercised, what you did, how you felt, and what you liked or didn't about the experience. As you continue to exercise, you will be able to track improvement and patterns, which will back you up with positive reinforcement that something is really changing in your body. Bonus: If you track it on an app and post it to social media, you will simultaneously be inspiring (or annoying, but whatever, haters gonna hate) to others and hold yourself accountable. If social media is not for you, record it in an exercise journal (on paper or online) and impress yourself. That's who you're doing this for, anyway, right?

Go. Get this done. Set your goals and smash them. You're one step closer to becoming who you've dreamed of being, one day at a time.

Chapter 7:
Stress and Self-Care

Two-week goal: Find methods that work for you to reduce your stress. Experiment with one, some, or all of the suggestions for self-care.

Are you a total stressball? Do your eyes fly open at 3:00 a.m. and you are as alert as if it were the middle of the day (hey, get your adrenals checked)? Do you take on way too many responsibilities? Do you overthink things?

In our fast-paced modern society, we seem to accept high levels of stress as a normal part of life. I speak with people of all walks of life in my practice and one of the questions that I ask the first time we sit down together is how stressed that individual feels. I suggest a scale (1-10) and they let me know the average range they are in on a weekly basis. To be honest, I don't hear a lot of people who consistently rate their stress level below a 5 out of 10.

This is not surprising when we consider the many things that are expected of us. Young people are stressed about finding a career that is going to pay enough to take care of what they want and need, about finding a good partner, and about paying off their massive debts. Parents of young families are bogged down with work, bills, raising children as best as they can, family issues, physical changes in their bodies as they walk farther and farther from being 25 years old, finances, saving for retirement, being able to give their children the best tools and preparation for life, being a good example, and juggling time for friendships, exercise, and healthy eating in the mix. Older adults whose children have flown out of the nest are concerned with their own physical health, the welfare of their children and grandchildren, the state of this crazy world, whether or not they will be able to make it financially as far as they need to, and whether or not they will be healthy and energetic enough to even enjoy retirement. Add in seasons of life when you are a caretaker for a family member, times of loss, hardship, job change, moving, serious illness and disease, and other challenges, and you've got a great big pile of stress all over the place.

This is a huge problem. (But don't like…stress about it. We're going to figure this out.)

There is a place for a proper amount of stress in your body. If you're meandering around the savannah on your African safari trip and a lion starts chasing you, you're going to be very glad for that "fight or flight" response to help you run faster (although, good luck, but still). When we are in danger, we need that influx of stress to push us physically to respond for our own survival. This is appropriate and acute stress. Unfortunately, we live in a society where chronic pervasive stress is the norm, and where having chronic stress is kind of like earning a badge for being tough and where some people almost like it.

Chronic stress creates havoc in every cell of your body. Your immune system is harmed, your hormone levels whack out, your metabolism changes, your ability to think clearly is hampered, and weird things can start happening to your body. Stress can manifest itself from hives, heart palpitations, tachycardia, inability to sleep, headaches, grinding your teeth, upset stomach, ringing in your ears, and many more. Emotionally, some people respond to their sense of losing control by an overwhelming desire to become a complete control freak, while others become extremely moody and agitated. For some people, it causes them to isolate themselves and feel worthless. You can lose focus on what you're supposed to be doing, become (even more) disorganized, procrastinate and avoid responsibility, make poor decisions, and be in a constant state of worry.

One of the things I ask each client after their stress level is how they deal with intense stress. I've heard a lot of different answers: sleep, drink, yell, freak out, exercise, work, polish the silver, lock myself away; but one of my favorite answers was from someone who said that the way that they deal with stress is to deal with the thing that is causing their stress and complete the things that are on the list of things to do. (Genius, really. Getting to the source of things and eliminating them, who would have thought of it?)

The consequences of long-term stress are serious and deadly. You may think it super fashionable now to never sleep, eat like junk, and work all the time, but living like this is a fast track to dying early. (Have you ever seen a picture of the warning sign that says, "Danger: Do not touch. Not only will this kill you, it will hurt the whole time you're dying."? That's basically how chronic stress will take you.) Heart attacks, stroke, obesity, hair loss, acne (did I hit your vanity button yet?), ulcerative colitis, Graves' disease, and on and on. Do me a favor and picture me grabbing your shoulders, looking straight into your eyeballs and telling you that you don't need this. Yes, you've got to do what you need to do, but you've also got to take care of yourself. There are ways of reducing the stress load that is in your life, and I want to help you to do that.

When you are going through a stressful time, I encourage you to practice self-care to pour back in to your body and mind and soul (and in some cases, your spirit). There are a few practices I want to share with you that you can choose from to help alleviate some of your stress and to take better care of yourself.

1. Saying no.

Oh, so weird, right? I know. Sometimes things can pile on fast. You're in the thick of it trying to be Superman or Wonder Woman, nailing this responsibility, checking this and that off of your to-do list, when another opportunity/responsibility/favor for a friend comes up, and you want to be that hero. You want to just tell yourself to suck it up and do the thing, because get real, you're not ever going to let anyone think that you're a selfish pig. But the problem is that you're barely keeping things afloat, you're not sleeping, you eat haphazardly, and you're chronically exhausted.

Repeat after me: It's okay to say no.

Even when it is something that might be fun, it's okay to say no. Even when a friend is asking, it's okay to say no. Even when it could get you more money, it's okay to say no. I would imagine that most people with the super stress complex going on are not those characterized by letting others down. You're usually the go-to person for everyone. You're capable and wonderful. If using a full-force "no" is difficult and painful, maybe you can practice saying, "not this time". You'd be amazed at how understanding people can be if you allow them the opportunity. Don't pile unnecessary things onto your list when you're chronically (or acutely) stressed out. Just say no. (Thanks, Mrs. Reagan.)

2. Hot towel scrub.

This idea is one that I learned through school at the Institute for Integrative Nutrition. Many people who have body image issues feel very differently after doing this exercise. It is a way to be thankful for the body you have, and to take specific and gentle care of it. It's the only shell you've got for this ride around the sun, so live in it well and take care of it.

The practice is to stand at your sink with a washcloth or a small towel that you've gotten wet with warm water. Some people find it beneficial to use essential oils to complement their overall experience and to help them relax even more. The warm cloth is placed on the skin (usually starting at the hands or wrists) and moved in small circles to enhance circulation. It is important to press firmly, but not so much that you're scraping your skin off and hurting yourself. It's enough to just wake your skin up and make it a little pink. You follow this up your arms, to your shoulders, neck, face, chest, stomach, back, legs, and down to your feet and toes. While you're doing this, just focus on relaxing your shoulders and breathing deeply, reminding yourself to chill out.

This relieves stress, opens your pores, activates your lymphatic system (as you massage your underarms and near your groin), and promotes circulation. It is a great practice right before bed as it is calming (and warming!). It is important to do this standing at the sink and not while showering, as I think that the difference in temperature between the air and the warm cloth makes for a shockingly good experience, rather than feeling like you're just washing your pits in the shower.

Clients who have body image issues have reported that this exercise made them involuntarily cry as they connected with their bodies. It was a vast change from often being unkind to their body to being sweet to it and taking care of it. Clients with bipolar and depressive symptoms also reported that this practice calmed them and made them feel more in balance.

It's free, what do you have to lose? Give it a try tonight before you go to bed and see if it works for you.

3. Essential oils to combat anxiety, pain, and depression[21]

I can hear some of your eyes rolling from here, but before you dismiss it as hocus pocus magic voodoo sauce, I want to share some of the scientific findings about various essential oils and their effects on stress, anxiety, pain, and depression. In 2008, a study was done with hospice patients where once a day for a week, they got a hand massage with a blend of essential oils (bergamot, frankincense, and lavender) and a carrier oil. 100% of the patients reported having less pain and less depression after just one week.[22] Not enough? In 2011, an experiment was done with elementary school teachers (who are known to work under constant stress). The teachers did an inhalation of bergamot essential oil for ten minutes. The results? Their blood pressure went down, their heart rates went down, and the rest of their autonomic nervous system activity moved toward a state of equilibrium.[23] In another animal study, mice received injections of bergamot oil (I'm not recommending you do that, I'm just highlighting an interesting point) that proved to be as effective as diazepam (valium). In 2007, a study found that lavender oil reduced serum cortisol levels in healthy (stressed out) men.[24]

We do not often question the pharmaceutical industry's solutions for anxiety, depression, and other mental stresses and disorders, but we are conditioned to overlook the power that is in nature that tends to work in parallel with our bodies. You are well aware that you can go to your physician and ask for an anti-anxiety drug, but if you've ever heard a commercial on the radio or television, you had to also listen to 30 seconds of speed reading through the side effects. Thankfully, unless you have a specific allergic reaction to something, side effects to essential oils are generally rare in a proper dose. There may be certain essential oils that could interfere with medication, so check with your doctor.

Lavender oil (lavender *L. angustifolia*) has been tested to treat general anxiety and has been as effective as the potentially addictive psychoactive drug benzodiazepine (lorazepam) in a six-week study when taken orally.[25] It did not have a sedative effect, and was well-tolerated, and the researchers found it to be a viable option instead of the pharmaceutical.

Essential oils are powerful and are not to be taken haphazardly or flippantly. Be aware of proper dosing, and whether something can be taken internally or whether an oil is to be inhaled, diffused, or applied topically. Various oils can have a burning sensation if they are not applied with carrier oils (jojoba oil, olive oil, coconut oil).

Essential oils like lavender, bergamot, ylang ylang, vetiver, rose, chamomile, frankincense, sandalwood, sweet orange, grapefruit, and geranium may help you to reduce stress, anxiety, and even pain.

4. Exercise

This is one of my favorite ways to reduce stress and cope with grief. When you exercise, your brain kicks out endorphins, the happy drug for your whole body. When you are under a great deal of stress, you can feel the effects of it in your body. Sometimes it feels like knots in your stomach, or a heightened sensation in your chest and arms, or otherwise. When you employ aerobic exercise, there is almost an immediate release of these feelings. For me, it is almost like an exchange of energy: the energy your body was using to produce stress feelings can be transferred over to your activity (swimming, running, biking, etc.) until you experience a sense of exhaustion and your whole body can quiet down.

Aerobic exercise is a mood-enhancer. Regular physical activity prepares your body to be more able to deal with difficulties and stressful situations. Find something you love and go do it. (See the chapter on exercise for more ideas and benefits.)

5. Taking a bath

Maybe this is just something helpful for me, but I wanted to share it. There is something about soaking down into hot water (with Epsom salt and essential oils especially) that not only reduce muscle stress (like from a challenging workout), but mental stress. It is an inexpensive but generously rewarding therapy that you could potentially do on a near daily basis. For many people, soaking in Epsom salt can also improve sleep and concentration because the magnesium in Epsom salts is uploaded to your body via your pores and promotes relaxation and good sleep.

6. Journaling

For some people, writing is a good output for their emotions. When there are burdens that you are carrying, and you can't keep it bottled up anymore, one of the things you can do to help process it and to express yourself is to journal. It is a creative outlet that helps you to say difficult things that you may not be comfortable saying. It also can help you to really see what it is you are feeling and why. Allowing these things to be said (without actually saying them to their intended recipient) may be a good way to discharge stress in difficult situations. (I am not suggesting this as a way to not deal with people directly in your life, but there are some times that it is not possible to do so: the person has died, you are no longer in contact with them, etc.) You can also use this exercise to release the initial anger or frustration so that when you do speak with them, you can think more clearly and use logic in your interaction.

7. Laughing

Laughing is one of my favorite things to do in the whole world. I value a great sense of humor as much as I do extreme intelligence, and I think with good reason: laughing reduces stress! Laughing releases endorphins, oxygenates your body, stimulates heart, lungs, and muscles. Laughter soothes tension through relaxation. It improves your immune system, helps you to relieve pain, and helps you to feel connected with others.

This may seem a little crazy, but you should try it anyway. Do you know that you can make yourself really laugh by starting off in fake laughter? I was at a health coaching conference for the Institute for Integrative Nutrition and Joshua Rosenthal was teaching about laughter and we did an exercise. Everyone started fake laughing and it sounded so absolutely ridiculous that the next thing you know, everyone was really laughing – and hard. It felt great and I recommend it. If you don't have any Monty Python or Seinfeld handy, this is a great option.

8. Praying

If you are not a person of faith, perhaps this seems strange to you to be included in a list of things to reduce stress and to be considered self-care. Many studies have been done that show the relationship between faith, spirituality, and a negative correlation between depression, anxiety, delinquency, and suicidal thoughts and behaviors.[26] It is not so surprising to connect these as faith gives people a sense of purpose, a hope, a connection with others, a connection to God, and a way to make sense of the world.

Psalm 9:9-10 says, "The LORD is a stronghold for the oppressed, a stronghold in times of trouble. And those who know your name put their trust in you, for you, O LORD, have not forsaken those who seek you." (English Standard Version)

Philippians 4:6-8 states, "[D]o not be anxious about anything, but in everything by prayer and supplication with thanksgiving let your requests be made known to God. And the peace of God, which surpasses all understanding, will guard your hearts and your minds in Christ Jesus. Finally, brothers, whatever is true, whatever is honorable, whatever is just, whatever is pure, whatever is lovely, whatever is commendable, if there is any excellence, if there is anything worthy of praise, think about these things." (English Standard Version)

Those are encouraging things to remember in the midst of stress and trouble, and the comfort that can be derived from these verses provides hope when things feel crazy.

9. Massage therapy or foam rolling

These are two other favorite ways to reduce stress. Massage therapy is much preferred to foam rolling because of human interaction and the benefit of touch, but foam rolling is a much more economical option. Studies have been done in regards to the stress-reducing effects of massage therapy (I'll volunteer. Pick me, pick me!). One study selected women going through one of the most stressful times of their lives: labor and delivery. Volunteers were selected to either use taught breathing exercises or massage therapy to help manage pain and stress. The women who received massage therapy had a better mood, less anxiety, less pain, shorter labors, a shorter hospital stay, and less postpartum depression![27]

Foam rolling is very physically effective in essentially being a meat tenderizer for your muscles. If your stress is carried in your muscles (neck, back), you may be able to treat the symptoms by rolling it out on the newest helpful torture device known as the foam roller. You'll laugh, you'll cry, but you'll feel much better when you're finished.

10. Having a cup of tea

Originally when I included this recommendation in the list of things you can do to reduce stress and take good care of yourself, I did it more from of the wisdom of my Grandma than from science. I was very close with my Grandma and she lived until the ripe old age of 101. She had a (multiple, actually) cup(s) of tea every single day of her life and she taught me to do the same. From a young age, I sat in her kitchen and she would put the kettle on the gas stove until it was whistling and then pour it over some black tea in a tea pot she saved for me to use. She would let me use a proper tea cup and saucer (not a barbaric mug) and pour in a little milk. Quite frankly, I think it is the only thing my Grandma ever drank (besides an occasional ginger ale). She had it with hamburgers as well as toast, out at restaurants, and in our homes. When she would receive stressful news or be worried about one of her children or grandchildren, she would say that she just needed a cup of tea. Upon that first sip, she would exhale and say, "Oooh, that's good!" It was like music to her soul. And if it wasn't nearly boiling hot, it was totally worthless.

I am so happy to find that science backs this up. I wish I could have told her this (she would not have been surprised *at all*), but since I can't share it with her, I'll tell you instead. In a double-blind placebo controlled experiment (The researchers are English. Tea shall not be trifled with.) over six weeks, it was found that tea drinkers' bodies came back to homeostasis after experiencing stress more quickly than non-tea drinkers[28]. Cortisol levels dropped more after the same amount of time, and blood platelet activation was lower in the tea drinkers (that is linked to blood clotting and heart attacks). This is great because chronic and pervasive stress is what kills us. Black tea pulls us back down to normal much more quickly, allowing us to spend less time in a heightened stressful state.

I write this today on her birthday, January 5. It should be a national holiday in honor of her and tea. Go have a cup and raise it up to Norah and a reduction to your stress levels.

Action steps

Over the next two weeks, it is likely that at some point you will experience some stress, if you are not already experiencing it chronically. Choose one or a few of these methods for self-care and see how they work for you. Take care of yourself. Treat your body with care. It's the only one you've got and when it's done, your game is over. Go out there and win.

Chapter 8:
Just Go To Sleep

Two-week goal: Get at least 7-8 hours of sleep a night. If that is impossible, try to get as many 7 to 8 hour night's sleep as you can.

Falling asleep at the kitchen table while working on the computer is a really great way to start off a chapter on sleep. Sleep, although pleasant to most, is an activity that most people find very difficult to be consistent with and to get sufficient amounts because of our very busy lives. I'm going to be really honest with you. Out of all the suggestions in this book, getting adequate sleep is the one thing that I struggle with most. I have just so many fabulous things I want to cram into my days that they often extend quite late into the night and I can't wait to wake up, leap out of bed, and start over again early the next day.

This is still stupid and a very bad idea. I'm going to be talking to myself throughout this chapter, so just bear with me. I had to be real with you on this before we even start, but this is not an excuse for you to say that since I have trouble with it, it's okay and you don't need to try. No. Unacceptable. Go for the best, no matter who joins you or doesn't. Which, by the way, I am trying to be conscious of this and make changes. As I write this chapter, it is nearing an appropriate bedtime, and I've set a time for shutdown so that I can go to sleep, even though I have five ridiculously interesting tabs open on sleep research and I'm so excited about it that my heart is pounding. Reading over some of the research is terrifying me enough to seriously start doing something about it on a consistent basis. Let's roll on this one together.

There are many reasons why we ought to try to get appropriate amounts of sleep (which, by the way is at least 7 hours, but depends on your age). Let me start off by telling you something a little disturbing – that is, a division of the World Health Organization (WHO) has determined that night shift work is a probable human carcinogen and puts you at risk for cardiovascular disease[29]. The research shows that a disruption in circadian rhythm of a subset of the population (namely, flight workers and night shift workers) had a significant increase in breast and prostate cancers. There is a theory that says this must have something to do with melatonin, but as of yet, the mechanisms are not exactly well-known. It is thought that it is linked to an increase in estrogen production (and high estrogen levels are related to various cancers).

There is an amazing process going on in your body that has to do with your circadian rhythm (*circadian* is Latin for "around a day") and with a chemical called adenosine. Adenosine builds up in your blood all day. The longer you are awake, the more of it your body has. The more that you have in your blood, the more tired you are. When you finally do go to sleep, your body starts the cleanup process and sweeps away the adenosine. Adenosine is responsible for widening blood vessels, giving you a steady heartbeat, and acts as a natural pain killer. If you do not get an appropriate amount of sleep and incur a sleep debt, you will never clear away your base adenosine levels (and that messes you up all over the board). Do you know what blocks the adenosine receptor? Caffeine. You're not surprised.

Melatonin is the other hormone that helps regulate your sleep. It is affected by light and is produced by the pineal gland in your brain. Melatonin starts its climb in the late afternoon, into the evening and night, and then drops off early in the morning as you're about to wake up. If you are a late shift nurse or someone else who works at night, it is especially important to help your body adjust to your sleep schedule by using light or darkness to help you wake or sleep. If you're coming home in the morning and the sun is up, you may want to wear sunglasses to help ease the transition into sleep when the world is waking up.

You may have heard people refer to "blue light". This is a very short wavelength. It is great for the daytime – it promotes alertness and mood – but it is very disruptive to your circadian rhythm when you're trying to go to sleep. Blue light is found in electronics (cell phones, laptops, TV screens) and in energy saving lightbulbs. It sends a signal to your brain that it is essentially high noon and it is time to rock it out. This may not bother you if you're staying up later to meet a deadline, but if you are in the habit of watching television before bed, you are sending your brain a very confusing signal. Have you ever plopped onto your couch, turned on the TV, and started watching, but found that even though you were quite exhausted, you were not falling asleep? It probably wasn't because the show was so exciting – it may be more likely that it is because it was messing with your biology. Maybe this is why you tell yourself at 10:30 you're going to bed after one more YouTube video but then find yourself watching strange how-to videos or German Shepherd dogs and lizards eating spaghetti at 2:45 in the morning while you roll over and ask yourself, "Why are you like this?!" Now you know, and knowing is half the battle.

If you get even an hour less per night of sleep than you ought to, you're falling into a sleep debt. Sleep debt accumulates, just like that credit card (or twelve) you have in your wallet. Not paying off either debt is going to cause you problems. A screwed up sleep pattern and a sleep debt are tied to obesity, cancer, diabetes, and heart disease. For people suffering from insomnia, the risk of depression and anxiety is *twenty times higher* than those who get an appropriate amount of sleep.[30] You have an increased risk of weight gain and obesity because two of your hunger hormones, ghrelin and leptin, are adjusted when you aren't getting adequate sleep.

Leptin is the hormone that suppresses hunger and ghrelin is the hormone that increases your appetite and is tied in to your body weight. When you don't get enough sleep, leptin tanks and ghrelin increases.[31] I suppose it only makes sense – if your body didn't get energy from you sleeping at night, maybe it will help you seek out energy by way of food. It is great that your body has a backup plan for when you failed to deliver what it needs, but it's not the most optimal way to go.

You will not be surprised to hear that a lack of sleep also has a negative effect on your mood. When you do not get appropriate amounts of sleep, you are irritable, short-tempered, and stressed out. That is because even a small decrease in sleep causes elevated levels of cortisol, your stress hormone.[32] You want to rest and digest, not to live in a state of fight or flight. You are more likely to yell at your spouse and children, forget things, injure yourself, and be an all-around world class jerkface. You have to be a very special person to successfully pull off classic jerkhood, so maybe you should just go lay down and spare the rest of us your wrath. People who got good sleep reported being able to handle the stressors of their day much easier than those who didn't.

Hey guys, one more thing for you – sleep disorders may reduce your testosterone levels.[33] Did you want a bro for your moobs, a big jiggly belly, an impaired libido, and erectile dysfunction? Just checking. Add that to the list of things to be grumpy about.

Let's just go over those amazing benefits of not getting a good night's sleep, shall we? Neglecting a proper sleep can:

- Put you at a much higher risk for breast and prostate cancer
- Increase your risk for heart disease
- Skyrocket your chances at obesity
- Push you toward diabetes
- Make you suffer from depression and anxiety
- Decrease testosterone levels in men
- Screw up your hunger hormones so you eat a lot more (ghrelin and leptin)
- Turn you into a jerky, yelling, forgetful, injured stressed mess (from increased cortisol levels)

Wow, sounds great.

Before we go any further, you need to know how much sleep you ought to be getting so you know what to aim for. According to the National Sleep Foundation, these are the optimal amounts of sleep for each age group.

Age	Optimal amount of sleep (in hours) in a 24-hour period
0-3 months old	14-17
4-11 months old	12-15
1-2 years old	11-14
3-5 years old	10-13
6-13 years old	9-11
14-17 years old	8-10
18-64 years old	7-9
65 years old +	7-8

Does that look like the amount of sleep you are currently getting? If not, we need to find some ways to help you improve your sleep hygiene.

1. Block the blue light.

I'm not suggesting that you must adopt an Amish lifestyle by using only candles and banishing your electronics, but there are tools that you can use to minimize the blaring blue light effect into your brain, ruining your circadian rhythm and throwing off your melatonin. The best thing would be to avoid electronic device usage right before bed, especially television. If you cannot avoid using your computer or phone (because you are working on something that can't wait), there are programs and apps that you can run that will switch your screen to a redder tone as the sun sets. While it is running, you cannot distinguish the difference, but your brain can. The program you can run on your computer is called f.lux and if you have an Android phone, you can download an app (I use Twilight) to avoid the negative effects of blue light at night. If you are an Apple user, you may already have a program built in that does this for your mobile device. Otherwise, if you want to set a trend, you can pick up some red/orange hued glasses and wear them around at night. People may sing the song to you, but you can use it as your opportunity to bring sleep hygiene awareness to all of your friends and family.

If you are willing to try, I recommend doing a 30-day experiment of removing the television from your bedroom. It will take you two minutes to unplug it and move it to a different room and, bonus - if you really hate it and miss it, it's not permanently gone. You have good sleep to gain, more connection with your family, more peaceful thoughts right before you go to bed, and a good example to set for your littles. You are much better served using the last few minutes before you go to bed to reflect on your day, set up your goals for the next, and to take a moment to be thankful for what you have. If you have difficulty getting the appropriate amount of sleep, this may go a long way in helping you to get where you need to be.

2. Avoid caffeine 4-6 hours before bedtime.

Some people swear that they can drink four cups of coffee an hour before bed and then hit the pillow and go right to sleep, while others are very sensitive to caffeine and can have their sleep significantly disrupted if they consume anything caffeinated after noon. Because we know that caffeine blocks the adenosine receptor (the hormone that makes you tired), it is not an exceptionally intelligent choice to make for your biology.

Caffeine is one of the main addictions that I deal with in my health coaching practice (second only to sugar) and it is not surprising that many people also have difficulty sleeping well and sleeping enough. I am not inherently against having any caffeine (I drink one cup of black tea every morning), but I think that the amount that we consume in our modern world is excessive. If you need more than two cups of coffee per day to function in your life, you have a problem. You are whipping your adrenals into a frenzy and making withdrawals from an account that you do not want to run out. Caffeine gives you that artificial boost, making it difficult (if not impossible) for you to be able to listen to your body's signals. Turn it down for sleep.

3. Be aware that alcohol before bed disrupts your sleep.

This is not to say that you should now become a day-drinker. Alcohol does not disrupt your circadian rhythm, but it alters your sleep by reducing your REM (rapid eye movement) sleep. When you drink alcohol in the evening, you are more likely to fall asleep more quickly, but in the latter half of your sleep to experience sleep disturbance and REM suppression.[34] REM sleep is vital because that is the stage of sleep that creates dreams, makes and retains memories, promotes learning, and increases brain activity. In studies, rats that were deprived of REM sleep lived significantly shorter lives.[35]

4. Be more concerned with setting a bedtime than an alarm for the morning.

The thought here is that you really need to make time to go to bed at an appropriate time. Make it an appointment like everything else you do in your day. Prioritize the things in your day so that you will accomplish what is most important so that you will be able to go to bed and give yourself enough time for sleep. It is important. It is your health, your happiness, and your wellbeing. It deserves a spot in the lineup and not to be put last on the list. (And then wake up in the morning and crush your goals.) If you are trying to prioritize your health, you need to prioritize getting yourself to bed at the right time. Nobody is going to make this happen for you, you have to do it yourself.

5. Work in parallel with your biology to help yourself to get to sleep.

Magnesium is an excellent supplement to help you get to sleep. Many people take it orally, but I prefer to soak it in via Epsom salt in a bath before I go to bed. After soaking in an Epsom salt bath, I have found that I have the deepest sleep. It's the magnesium.

Otherwise, lavender essential oil can be used (via inhalation or combined with a carrier oil and used topically) to help promote relaxation and sleep.

Melatonin is the go-to for people suffering from occasional insomnia. Melatonin is sold as a supplement, but you can also consume certain foods to boost melatonin. The food will not cross into your brain, but when it hits your gut, your gut can signal up to your brain (I love the microbiome-gut-brain axis!). The food with the most melatonin (by a long shot) is tart cherry juice concentrate. Sweet cherries are tasty but very useless in this regard, so if you want to go this route, please make sure you are getting the correct cherry. (Tart cherry also reduces inflammation and has helped many of my clients with osteoarthritis.) Otherwise, other foods with melatonin are walnuts, mustard seed, corn, rice, ginger root, peanuts, and barley grains.

6. Exercise, but not right before bed.

Besides Epsom salt baths, the best sleep I ever have are the nights after I sprint for five miles. It works every time. You don't have to do exactly that, but getting good exercise is a quality way to help your body to sleep and relax later in the evening. If you exercise right before bed, you are likely to be really fired up and not able to sleep (especially if your volleyball teammate just served 25 times in a row and you're so excited from that massive win that you could climb a mountain with your adrenaline).

Waking up at night

If you have ever had the delightful experience of having your eyes fly wide open for no apparent reason at 3:00 in the morning, you will know that it can mess you up pretty well. You want to be asleep, but for reasons unbeknownst to you, you have been thrust into a two-coffee level of wakefulness like a switch was thrown in your brain. You may think, "Why can't I feel this awake when my alarm goes off?" Or, if you're like me, you think, "Oh no! I'm awake. It's bad to be awake at this time. Go to sleep." And then you think about going to sleep so much that you can't sleep. "I said, 'GO TO SLEEP!'" But your brain doesn't listen to you, and instead it starts freaking out because now you *can't* sleep.

So you now have a completely irrational 3:00 a.m. conversation in your head going on that is promoting unnecessary levels of stress and you can feel your heart just pounding and your blood sprinting through your veins. (That's usually the point I disdainfully ask, "Why are you like this?")

If I am remembering at all that I can be rational (even though it's 3:00 in the morning and I'm going through a grocery list and planning which days I'm going to go running and how better to save the world), I will remind myself that I can transition myself from stress to rest and digest by employing a good "belly breathing" technique.

It takes barely any thinking. I breathe in for four seconds, filling up my belly (not my chest), hold for four seconds, breathe out for four seconds and repeat. Even if you do this just a few times, you can force your body to calm down. (I SAID, "CALM DOWN!") This exercise can be utilized at any point in the day when you feel like your stress levels are freaking you out. It's better than resorting to the throat punch (and by a significant margin).

Side note: If you consistently wake up at 3:00 in the morning, you may need to have your adrenal function checked. Consistently waking at that time is a sign of adrenal fatigue. Severe adrenal fatigue was best described by one of my clients who said that adrenal fatigue was so debilitating that if there were to be a fire in her house, she would not have the energy to get up and walk out. Do not push your body to that point. It will yell louder and louder at you until you listen or until it shuts you down.

Action steps

Over the next couple weeks, set a bedtime so that you are getting an appropriate amount of sleep. Remove the television from your bedroom and avoid the blue light. Be aware of your caffeine and alcohol intake and how that affects your sleep quantity and quality. If you have trouble sleeping, try lavender, magnesium, tart cherry juice concentrate, Epsom salt baths, or something else that helps you relax. Make a bedtime ritual – it works for toddlers; it can work for you. Get the sleep you need and stop making excuses. It's important. Go write down your sleep goals and make it happen, starting tonight. If you wake up at 3:00 in the morning, think of something lovely, and do your belly breathing until you go back to sleep.

Goodnight and happy dreams.

Note: Since the writing of this chapter, I have thought a lot about getting proper sleep. I have successfully accomplished making a routine of a more appropriate bedtime. What worked for me was setting my bedtime as if it were an appointment, and just making myself go to bed when the time came. (It is both as simple and as complicated as that.) It really is important for your overall health and happiness to get proper sleep and you are not a hero if you destroy yourself in this area. You are just performing at less than your best. When you can get the sleep you need, you will be sharper to attack the projects on your plate, getting them done with a fresh, happy, and healthy brain. It's almost as if you're adding productivity. (Plus, you'll swim faster. So just listen to me and do it. Okay? Thanks. Glad we had this talk. Suck it up, buttercup, just do it. Excuses? No thanks. I don't want to hear them. I only say this because I care.)

Chapter 9: Laughter and Positive Attitude

Two-week goal: Over the next few weeks, find things to be grateful for, laugh, and kick negative thoughts to the curb

Maybe you find it odd that a chapter on laughter and a positive attitude is included on a book for overall health. Well, that's because you're a total grump. Time for a change, bucko. Get on the bus, it's leaving.

I love to laugh. I may verge on the obnoxious when I participate in things that make me laugh, but I relish the ability to suck the life out of life, and I think that in this area not only is there no exception, but it is one that I want to push the limits and enjoy most. My favorite people in the whole world are people who can make me laugh. Remember what Marilyn

Monroe had to say about laughter – "If you can make a girl laugh, you can make her do anything." (I mean, not *anything*. I'm not touching high fructose corn syrup with a ten-foot pole, even if you're Jimmy Fallon, John Cleese, Colleen Ballinger, Tina Fey, and Lilly Singh all put together.)

This aspect of life is so important to me that I thought it vital to include in my business motto, "Get healthy, be happy." If you ask anybody what they really want out of life, you are likely to hear most people have an answer that really just boils down to being happy. We're not guaranteed happiness in this life, and those times that are most difficult produce the most character in us, but the shards of joy we can find sprinkled throughout are dear and precious and we ought to gobble them up as much as possible. When you are in the midst of the lowest times of life and you don't know how you're going to keep going because the waves are crashing over you, making you unable to breathe as the weight of your situation crushes your chest and sucks the life out of you, this is precisely when you need to find the small things in life to be thankful for and to find a few moments to laugh.

You will be very relieved to know that according to Dr. William Strean, in prescribing laughter to patients, there "are no substantial concerns with respect to dose, side effects, or allergies."[36] I hope someone was paid a lot of money to research that.

Before we go on, I just want to tell you something important. Two atoms were walking down the street when one cried out, "You stole an electron from me!"

Shocked and a little offended at the accusation, the second atom replied, "Are you sure?"

The first inhaled sharply in indignation, "I'm positive!"

Moving right along. (So good, right? I know!)

What are the benefits of laughter?

    1.   Increased immune response

Your immune system is on the job nonstop. It protects you from invaders that seek to destroy your health. The malicious itty bitties are thwarted by the army that is your immune system. They are the good guys who concern themselves with making sure you don't catch every cold, germ, and even fend off disease. Help them out. Besides taking a probiotic supplement and eating probiotic foods, give them a boost by laughing.

Stress is associated with a decreased immune function. The microbiome-gut-brain axis is absolutely fascinating. The health of your gut is a determinant of your mental health and vice versa. There is two-way communication between the little guys fighting in your intestines and your neurons. Give them a hand and find something to laugh about.

You know what? One time I had a really bad haircut. It was just awful! I hate to admit this, but after a while, it grew on me.

2. Decreased blood sugar levels

Diabetes is on the rise. In 1980, 108 million people suffered from diabetes, but by 2014, 422 million people were dealing with this disease. Type II diabetes can be significantly eradicated by lifestyle modifications – exercising, not smoking, eating food that is really food and not chemicals. This is not something you want to mess with. Diabetes causes blindness, kidney failure, heart attacks, stroke, and lower limb amputation.

A study was done wherein people with diabetes ate a meal and then afterwards listened to a lecture. The researchers then measured their insulin levels. They were all invited back the next day, ate the same meal again, but this time, instead of listening to a lecture, they watched a comedy. After watching the comedy, their blood sugar levels were lower than they were the first day![37]

If you are suffering from diabetes, I absolutely suggest that you find ways to laugh, but I also encourage you to make necessary lifestyle changes to make yourself feel better and to get out from under that diagnosis. Are you drinking soda? No, you're not anymore. You're done with that junk. Are you eating food that doesn't grow out of the earth or walk around on legs (fast food does not count, no matter how much you tell me you're eating the salad.)? Nope, quit that, too. I'm not going to mince words about it. You're on a path of destruction and I don't want you to die, go blind, or lose your feet. You have a lot to give to your family, friends, and this world. Get up and do something about it. Be an example. Be a remarkable story. You have it in you. Fight like you mean it. And laugh while you're at it. (This concludes my tirade. Now back to your regularly scheduled reading.)

By the way, what do you call a pig that is really into karate? Pork chop.

3. Better blood flow

A study done by the University of Maryland tested the effects of laughter on blood flow. Laughter causes the endothelial layer to dilate and expand, causing better blood flow. This is important because constriction of blood vessels is a factor in cardiovascular disease. The benefits they saw were equivalent of aerobic activity.[38] (This does not mean that you get to give up your morning swim because you're watching Billy Madison later, but it's still an amazing fact.)

According to the World Health Organization, cardiovascular disease is the number one cause of death globally. In 2012, cardiovascular disease took the lives of 17.5 million people, accounting for 31% of all global deaths. There are many factors that contribute to ill cardiovascular health, and this simple behavior modification stands to reduce blood vessel constriction. Your soul is happy when you laugh, and so is your heart.

Hey, did you hear what happened when the butcher backed up into his meat grinder? He got a little behind in his work.

4. Significantly increased pain tolerance

There are many pains associated with this life. Why not knock off a few wimp points by increasing your pain tolerance through laughter? Oxford University found that laughter elicited an endorphin-mediated opiate effect, and it was actually laughter (and not the feeling of happiness, or the being part of a group laughing, or any other factors outside of the laughter itself) that caused the study participants to be able to tolerate significantly higher levels of pain.[39]

I thought this study was amusing and interesting especially because the researchers took such care to make sure that it was actually laughter (and not being part of a group or the feeling of happiness) that was what caused an increase in pain tolerance. They recorded the study participants and their laughter and put them into situations of non-humor and humor and then tested them by squeezing their arms in a blood-pressure cuff, telling them to signal when they couldn't stand the pain anymore. After being in a situation where the participants were laughing, their pain tolerance significantly increased. This is amazing because laugher elicits an opiate effect!

I tried to test this just last night as I played volleyball when I responded to a vicious serve by setting the ball. (What was I thinking? I'm not sure. It was too high for a controlled pass and I did it out of reaction.) Both of my thumbs instantly jammed up and I started sweating from pain. I remembered this research and decided that I needed to experiment on myself. I employed moderately obnoxious behavior in an attempt to encourage my teammates toward hilarity (which was successful), causing myself to laugh, while I monitored my pain. It steadily decreased over the course of the game. I know that this is a single incidence, but I thought I would try it out as it cost me nothing and I only risked benefits. Next time you're injured, you could try it and see how it works for you. After all, Dr. Strean says there aren't any negative side-effects, so you may as well give it a chance.

Just wondering, but did you hear about those new corduroy pillows? They're making headlines!

5. Humor shows that you've won

One of the psychological supports of humor is that it shows that you've triumphed over pain, suffering, and a negative situation. There is a story of Freud that perfectly exemplifies this. As Germany annexed Austria, Freud was permitted to emigrate to England upon a written admission that he was not mistreated by the Nazis. His well-known, humorous, and sarcastic post script was, "I can heartily recommend the Gestapo to anyone."

After coming out on the other side of a difficult situation, humor allows you to be the winner. You were not taken down permanently by your trouble, you were not completely undone. In redressing your situation with humor, you stand triumphant over it, nearly mocking it and its attempt to disable you, while pushing it down beneath you. In employing humor, you beat the situation and show that it has not destroyed you.

Think of the many awful life situations that turn people toward bitterness, spewing acidic rancor in every direction. Anyone around them can see that they have been tainted by and made subject to their situation. Choose to grow over the top of it, pull through to the other side, and stand over it victorious.

You know, something strange happened to me this morning. I bought a new pair of shoes from a drug dealer. I don't know what he laced them with, but I've been tripping all day.

On my worst days, when things are so stressful and feel so awful, when things are not going the way I want them to and I can't take it anymore, I purposely make myself watch something funny for a few minutes before I go to bed. Recently I was having an exceptionally stressful and sad day, and I was up too late writing when I really wanted to wind down from a long week. I was feeling grumpy, cold, and sad, and it was midnight. I took a deep breath and decided I wasn't going to go to bed feeling like this. That's when I pulled out my favorite YouTube people and within minutes, found myself belly laughing. I was much happier and less stressed out when I went to bed. (The next morning I may have been accused of waking people up from laughing so much, but we all got over it.) I highly recommend it.

Positive Attitude

Besides laughter being a great medicine for your soul and body, having a positive attitude is a huge plus when you're facing this crazy life. Being an optimist has benefits and is explained in this way:

"Optimistic individuals are positive about events in daily life. In the research carried out regarding this perspective, positive correlations have been found between optimism and physical/mental well-being. Optimistic subjects tend to have more frequently protective attitudes, are more resilient to stress and are inclined to use more appropriate coping strategies.

...optimism, [is] characterized by the tendency to believe that negative events are inconstant (the negative event will not repeat itself), external (I am not responsible for the event) and specific (the event is 'specific', self-limiting and will not influence any other activities of mine and my life). Optimists believe that positive events are more stable and frequent than negative ones. They think that they can avoid problems in daily life and prevent them from happening, and therefore they cope with stressful situations more successfully than pessimists."[40]

Optimism correlates with positive mental and physical health. It is not a stretch to see how optimism and believing the best lends toward a positive mental state, but that it correlates with positive in the physical is something that we ought to be paying more attention to. In our western mindset, we discount much of how our thoughts and our spirits impact our bodies because we only consider the empirical to be legitimate. Great news for you, my western thinker: science backs it up. You can imagine that people with an optimistic outlook experience thoughts that the future will be positive, have less suicidal thoughts, display hope, and have strategies for dealing with problems when the arise. This contributes to a better quality of life.

The role that optimism plays in the physical is less known, although research is available. In a study on adults aged 65-85, a disposition of optimism predicted less probability of death by all causes, but especially and specifically cardiovascular death.[41] (That is great news since cardiovascular death is the number one cause of death globally. If you can dodge that bullet, you've missed a big one.) Even in cases of those who had atherosclerosis, their disease progressed more slowly when they had an optimistic disposition compared to those with a pessimistic outlook. Certain cancers have a significantly higher survival rate when a person is optimistic.[42]

Perhaps you are a naturally optimistic person and you are rejoicing over this information (as you should, and really, is anyone surprised that you're rejoicing at something?). Optimism is good for your mental and physical health. You stand to live a longer life as a result of your optimism. My 101-year-old Grandma said the secret to her long life was, "tea and being happy". Take a note from Norah, my dears. It's worth it to see the silver lining in things.

What if you're not naturally an optimist? One of the things that I say to my clients is that you need to talk to yourself instead of listen to yourself. We have this voice inside that can crop up and tell you lots of horrible things about yourself – you're not good enough, you aren't smart, you can't do it, people are looking at you thinking you're weird, you won't succeed, you probably won't get that job, your hair is too green, your voice is too quiet, everyone is skinnier than you, you can't achieve those dreams. Those things aren't very nice. What if that voice was talking to your dearest friend that way; what would you say?

You would likely tell it that it is wrong, and unkind, and to go away. The ironic thing is that you've never thought to stand up for yourself in your own head. It's your territory in there. Who has the right to come in and muck it up like that? Are you good with that? Kick it to the curb. You don't need to listen to that.

Speak kindly to yourself like you're a friend. When you hear one of those things pop up, stand up for yourself. Argue with it and put the smack down on it. When it tells you that you can't do it, you say that you can – and you will. You're going to be the best darn water-skier (or whatever it is) in the whole lake. You're going to get that job. You're going to rock your presentation. You're going to be efficient and get things done and change the world. Why not? Other people can do it and they're not better than you! Pull up that desire and go after it.

Many of my clients hear the negative voices of their parents repeating in their heads. Kick that out. You're an adult. Yes, it's crap that those things happened and you didn't get the reassurance and positive words that you needed when you needed them. Look at it from an adult perspective now. They screwed up (hopefully not on purpose – everyone has their own issues, right? Even if they did, you get to choose what lives in your head.), but you don't have to eat that up for the rest of your life. If you were standing there and heard a parent berating their child with the words that you've heard in your own head, what would you think – would you think that that child needed to hear that? That they should grab onto that and roll with it for the rest of their lives? Some of you are bold enough to step in and confront someone in a situation like that, but yet you allow that voice of the past to beat yourself up. Stand up for that little girl or boy that was you and shut it down. Make the decision to get rid of it.

Start speaking to yourself instead. Argue with that voice. Wake up in the morning, look at yourself in the mirror and say what you need to hear. I can do this. It's going to be a good day. Everything is going to work out just fine. I will do my best and the presentation and smile and I know people will like me and listen to me. I will be confident today. I am going to PR my race. I can swim a 100 fly and I'm going to give it my all. I can change the world!

When things don't fall the way that you want, you course correct. You don't throw yourself under the bus and give up. There's no use for junk talk. "See! I knew you were no good! What was the point in even trying! You *failure*!" What is that? Honestly. That does you no good. Instead, you take a look at things and say, "Well, that didn't work out. I didn't get that job, but you know what? It wasn't for me. Something better is out there. I can't wait to see what it is. I'm going to keep hustling and make it happen."

My life quote is, "I never lose. I win or I learn." It's all in the perspective. If things didn't work out the way you wanted them to, that does not mean it was necessarily your fault. It does not mean the world is against you. It does not mean that you will now fail at everything else. It does not mean that you are worth less because of it. It just means it didn't work out. That's it. It wasn't for you. Accept that something better is out there. Maybe not today, maybe not tomorrow, but if you've got your head on straight and you're working hard and taking care of things with your shiny new positive attitude, things have a tendency to line up just fine.

If you have trouble with this, there are a couple of exercises that you can do to help foster thinking toward the positive. The first thing is to journal daily on things that you are thankful for. Get a journal that you can write in at night before you go to bed. Put it by your bed and use your favorite pen. Give yourself just five minutes (or more, if you want) to write down a few things from your day that were good and that went well. Sometimes you might have to dig deeper than others, but something good is always there.

Find the beauty in the common. Enjoy the little things in life. Relish that hot cup of tea in the morning. Be thankful for friends or family who reach out to you or who you could call in a time of trouble. Be thankful that winter doesn't last forever, and when it feels like the clouds will never end, you know that spring will be even sweeter this year. Be grateful that you've met interesting people in your life and loved big. Be happy that you can transport yourself to jolly old Elizabethan England in the time of the larger than life monarchs through reading Alison Weir's fantastic novels. Be grateful that you can learn amazing things and expand your world inside your own mind.

The other exercise is related, but it encompasses things that you enjoy whether or not you got to experience them that day or not. It helps you to reflect and think about the grand and the simple pleasures of life that are specific to you and to what you love and to what sparks joy in your own heart. Write a list of 100 things that make you happy. Go back to that list when you are feeling like the world is dumping on you and remember that life is not all that bad. Some people died this morning and their story is over. (Yes, when you're really sad, you wish you could trade with them, but I want you here. Pain is temporary. You can get through.) If you've got breath in your lungs, be thankful, my dears.

I wanted to share my 100 things that make me happy list with you to give you ideas (and really just to show you just how weird I really am). Maybe some will resonate with you, but you have your own unique set of things and I encourage you to explore them and write them out. When I think of the things that make me happy, I wanted to make sure that I wasn't focusing on a lot of things that have a price tag on them. Our lives can be so full and rich even if we aren't (perhaps *especially* if we aren't) and enjoying the things that are all around us is part of finding joy in everyday life.

100 Things That Make Me Happy

1. A hot bath right before bed.
2. Seeing your kid swinging happily on the swing when they don't know you're watching.

3. The one cup of hot black tea you have at breakfast.
4. Laying with eyes closed in the sunshine.
5. Having a conversation and a cup of tea with someone who makes you so deliriously happy.
6. Being in the middle of an amazing book.
7. Speaking to someone in another language.
8. Hitting the bullseye on the first try.
9. When your favorite flavor of Kevita (water kefir) is available and on sale.
10. Oboro low smoke incense.
11. Smelling something that flashes you back to a moment in your life and it's so real, you can see and feel it.
12. When you must do the laundry and the basement is cold, but you can wrap a large hot towel around yourself and stick your head into the dryer and take a pretend nap on the warm clothes.
13. Finally sitting down after being on your feet all day.
14. What your kitchen/fridge/house/bathroom/vehicle looks like when it is perfectly clean.
15. Cracking an egg into a butter-filled cast iron pan that is so fresh, it's still warm.
16. Jumping into the pool (or a lake) and watching the bubbles rise up around you.
17. Staring at the sky in the middle of the summer at sunset floating on your back in the middle of a lake.
18. Showering outside.
19. Finishing a triathlon.
20. The lateness of sunset in the summer.
21. Walking barefoot in the grass when it's warm.
22. Hopping fences.
23. Cartwheels.
24. Getting paid to do what you thrive on.
25. The feeling right when the plane lifts off of the ground.
26. Sleeping until you wake up on your own.
27. New York City.
28. Having a passionate intellectual argument.
29. Laughing until you can't breathe.
30. Falling asleep with the window open.
31. Being able to fix something for someone.
32. Saunas.
33. The feeling of an amazing foot massage.

34. Falling asleep when you are exhausted.
35. Getting a package in the mail.
36. Writing with a black Bic gel ink pen in bold 1.0. (Since I wrote this, I've also come to love 0.7 gel ink pens. I'm not discriminating.)
37. Writing (or reading) a poem that expresses exactly where you are at that moment.
38. When herbs first sprout in tiny pots on your windowsill.
39. Digging your toes in the sand at the beach and not having anything requiring your immediate attention.
40. Getting a hug when you really needed one.
41. Lying in bed and realizing you got everything done you needed to that day.
42. Driving really fast (safely, of course).
43. Going for a run that exhausts your body, clears your mind, and alleviates your soul.
44. Painting your nails your favorite color.
45. Being alone in your own space.
46. Having a happy dream that when you wake up, it seems like it might really have happened.
47. Getting a text that makes you burst into laughter.
48. Re-reading a sweet message that makes you sigh happily.
49. Watching your itty bitties sleep.
50. Seeing the sunrise from the woods.
51. The memory of epic youthful shenanigans.
52. Mission Peninsula.
53. Being genuinely happy for someone else's good news.
54. Homemade bread with grass-fed butter.
55. Butter in general.
56. Being the person that someone wants to tell their new news to.
57. Your favorite classical/jazz music piece.
58. Finding the perfect gift for someone.
59. When it's been raining all day and then the sun peeks out brilliantly and overpoweringly.
60. Getting to see ancient art in person (and wondering how many eyes and generations across the whole world have taken in that same painting/sculpture).
61. Really great foodie-grade (dark, obviously) chocolate.
62. The mountains.
63. The first day that it feels like summer of the year.

64. Seeing a hummingbird.
65. Bohemian Rhapsody by Queen.
66. The scent of your favorite people.
67. Looking at your friend and knowing exactly what they're thinking at that moment.
68. PR-ing a race.
69. The silence, the vastness, the slowed movement, the feeling of anti-gravity, and the freedom of swimming underwater.
70. New running shoes, a new endurance suit.
71. A good hair day.
72. Teaching someone something and getting to watch the light bulb turn on in their head.
73. Delicious, wonderful, amazing, hippie-scented lotion.
74. Your favorite undies.
75. Finding someone who understands you.
76. An exceptionally beautiful face with mesmerizing eyes.
77. The vibrant green-ness of the grass in spring.
78. Campfires, fireplaces.
79. A hot washcloth covering your whole face.
80. Knowing that life usually works out just fine.
81. Learning.
82. Daisies and tulips.
83. Running past apple blossom trees in full bloom.
84. Seeing good friends again from a lifetime ago.
85. Summer + live music + being outside + your favorite drink
86. Orion in the night/early morning sky.
87. Buffalo meat.
88. Listening to somebody's story.
89. Flying down a hill full speed on your bike.
90. Getting a massage when you are so sore that you involuntarily cry-laugh-drool-gasp in reaction to muscle pressure. Stop! No, go. Stop! Go! Ow! More!
91. Getting in a(n outside) hot tub after skiing (or swimming/running/biking) especially while it is snowing.
92. The first red, ripe, garden tomato of the season.
93. Icelandic full-fat yogurt.
94. Getting into a bed of just-washed sheets and a super fluffy down comforter.
95. Falling asleep to your hair being played with.
96. Night swimming.

97. Listening to your little one laugh ridiculously at something ridiculous.
98. The way Londoners speak.
99. Kitchen dancing.
100. The thought that you can change the world for the better a little bit every day.

Action steps

Talk to yourself, don't listen to yourself. Write out the positive and speak it daily. Write out what you're thankful for. Make a list of 100 things that make you happy. It is good for your health, your heart, and promotes longevity.

You're wanted, you're loved, and you're worth it. You have a purpose here and the world needs you. This life is not haphazard nonsense, and although it is sometimes chaotic, it is a beautiful tapestry. Embrace it. Find your spot and make a difference.

Chapter 10: Organization

Two-week goal: Tackle a space and make it work for you

You may be wondering why on earth I'd include a chapter on organization in a book about overall health. It may be because I feel a strong affinity for those who organize like they're trying to win some kind of OCD award, or because I believe that the environment of your home, office, desktop, closets, refrigerator, cupboards, and car are a reflection of the inside of your brain. (Okay, both.) It affects your mental health and your stress level, and that has a strong influence on your physical health and wellbeing.

Organization is something near and dear to my heart. My mother tells me that before I was two years old, I was lining my shoes up next to each other in perfect alignment in my closet. As a child, I would invade my lifelong friend's room and clean it up for her (Incidentally, we were college roommates and I made her bed for her on a daily basis. We agreed on one section of the room that could be an untouchable mess. Thanks for putting up with me, Lyndi.). When I was a teacher, I marked the tiles so that the desks were evenly spaced in rows and would dismiss students from class when their rows were re-straightened. Milk, eggs, bread, yogurt, and veggies have assigned seating in my refrigerator (I mean, obviously, right?). My clothes hang in my closet based on clothing type, and then within each section they are arranged by color: dark to light (this is easy since I only wear 5 colors – black, grey/silver, navy/blue, pink, white).

It was very natural for me to become a professional organizer with all of this going on. I owned my own organizational business with the determination to help people who wanted to make efficient systems within their homes or offices. (Remember the TV shows where the people would go in and make people throw a bunch of things away and then reorganize what was left? That was essentially what I did.) When there is significant disorganization, it is challenging for things to be highly productive because there is an increased difficulty with finding necessary things. Much time is wasted in completing a task because time and energy are spent trying to locate items.

With many people, but especially busy professionals and moms, when your eyes land in various locations around your home, you are reminded of and collecting a to-do list with everything you see. A basket of laundry that isn't yet folded on the couch, a pile of dishes waiting to be washed, a stack of papers on the desk that need to be filed and dealt with, and whatever else surrounds you reminds you of things that you need to accomplish but haven't. This discrepancy of things needing to be accomplished but aren't leads to increased stress as you feel overwhelmed in your own space.

I firmly believe that your environment is a reflection of the inside of your mind. If you can take control of what is outside, you can in some way calm what is going on inside. (I do not say this as a way to avoid feelings that need to be dealt with, but as a help for you to reduce stress in life.) Imagine the difference in walking in to your own space where everything is accomplished, clean, and in a good working order. You feel that you are ahead of things and able to master the tasks that will face you that day. You already have things checked off of your to-do list and you are fresh. This is what I want you to feel. I want you to have success and I want you to feel that you can conquer your day head on, prepared, and equipped. I also want for your space to be a place of peace and sanctuary for you, a place that you look forward to being where you can recharge and feel renewed.

The United States is a country of excess. The majority live above their means and have far more things than needed. If you have never travelled to a less-developed country and come back with fresh eyes for what you've got, I highly recommend the experience if you're ever able to take it. I went to El Salvador a couple times for mission work and was ashamed of my excess when I saw that the sweet women I was working with had two pair of underwear: one to wear and one to wash and hang out to dry for the next day. I determined to try to hold that ideal as best as possible but to function reasonably within this society upon my return.

If you have far too many things, you have an insurmountable task of getting organized. It is not possible to look and feel organized when you can't walk through your rooms because you have so many things. It is not cute (nor is it safe) to stack your boxes to the ceiling, perhaps attempting to replicate a creative supermarket beer display. I'm going to tell you something difficult, but you need to hear it. If you have more stuff than you know what to do with, you need to get rid of some things. You must part with the things that are holding you back and holding you down. They are heavy and weigh on you mentally.

Everything you own costs you something. It should be giving back to you as well. It costs your space. It costs your care and your energy – dusting it, washing it, moving it, packing it. If it is not significantly giving back to you and "sparking joy" (the words of world-renowned Japanese organizational guru, Marie Kondo), you should consider if it deserves to keep taking from you.

One question I always asked my organizational clients when we began a project to organize a space was, "If I came and waved a magic wand and everything disappeared from this area, what would you miss and regret that it was gone?" This gets straight to the heart of things. This reveals to you what is truly necessary. The rest is negotiable.

The second question is more revealing and one I want you to ask yourself: How would you feel if it were all gone? I cannot express to you the amount of times people looked at me and their gut reaction response was that they would feel overwhelmingly relieved. If this is the case, I want to ask you what is holding you back!

You are forgetting that you really can make change. You do not have to do things just because you've always done them or because that's the way everyone around you does them. You are not stuck. This is your life. Do something about it. Why are you holding yourself back?

Here are some things you can do to help clear your space and make your life work more efficiently:

1. Make your bed every single day.

This is a serious Martha Stewart-ism. Your bed takes up so much eye space in your bedroom (unless you have a gigantic bedroom that's the size of a ballroom, and if you do, you probably have your butler make your bed for you anyway, so never mind) that it can make a significant difference in the look of the overall organization of that space just by doing this simple thing. It is obviously preferable for you to do this in the morning just after waking up so that you can enjoy the visual benefits all day. Accomplishing anything straight away in the morning is a plus to get you going toward myriads of productivity throughout the day, so once you have that checked off your to-do list, there's no telling what you'll be able to do. This also helps you to avoid meandering back into your room, flopping down fully into bed and pulling the covers over your face to avoid the day.

Make your bedroom your sanctuary, a place where you can go and truly relax and rest. If you have at least one space that is organized and beautiful, you can feel more at peace when the stress of the world crashes down upon you.

2. Put things back where they belong the first time.

I know that this is not always practical (think: entering your home after the grocery store, determined that you were only going to make one trip so your arms are lined with twelve grocery bags, a purse, the mail, a phone on your ear, and a water bottle precariously balancing while you unlock your door), but as much as you are able to put this into practice, the more time you will eventually save in life. It only stands to reason – if you've set something down in a location that is not its home, you'll have to move it again in the near future to its home. You just made two actions for one object. How many times do you do that throughout the day? Setting it down where it doesn't belong clutters that area and puts something else on your future to-do list.

3. Assign things their own "home" in your space.

Did you read this point and furrow your brows? Yes, it's true. I believe that *everything* you own should have a home. If you haven't got enough space for everything to have a home, you either have too many things or not enough space. (It's usually the former.) Think about how and where you use the item to determine the most logical location for each thing. It is a waste of time if you always have to walk across your kitchen to get your pots and pans and bring them back to the stove, or if you have to hike across the room to put your silverware back after washing it. If possible, put items where they can be most useful to you.

If you notice that you have run out of places to put things, then you have run in to the perfect opportunity to purge. Space and money are commodities with similar characteristics. Do you have sufficient funds? Then you can (potentially) buy something. If you do not, then you should not. Do you have sufficient space? Then you can keep that thing. If you do not, then you should not. If you want to keep something, you need to get rid of something else. It's practically revolutionary.

4. Purge.

Start by asking yourself what are the most important things in a space and what you would miss if the whole room vanished. Work with that in mind. Sometimes you have to be in a little bit of a ruthless mood to be exceptionally successful at purging (may I suggest a soundtrack of rap music?). If you're going in to purging with lovey feelings about all of your sentimental objects, you're not going to get very far. Put on your game face and make things happen. If you have something that is sentimental but you also have a little voice in the back of your head that wants to get rid of it, you can take a picture of it and save it that way. If it's main use to you is something that is just sentimental, then perhaps you should let the physical go and hold the emotional. Otherwise, you're being held captive by your stuff.

When you go through your things, make three piles: keep, get rid of/donate, and an "I just can't do it" pile. If there is something that you can't deal with, put it in a box. Seal the box. Pack the box away. Write a note on it with a date telling you that if you don't use anything in the box before then, it is time. Aim for six months to a year. If you don't open it in that time, its fate has been decided. Do not open it. You will be tempted to keep everything if you do. Carry it (or have someone else do it for you if you'll be too tempted) out to the curb and kiss it goodbye. Its time with you has ended. It had its place in your journey and now let that baby grow wings and fly away. Give yourself the gift of letting things go and being free.

In my time as a professional organizer, I found that there were a few common things that many clients kept around the house "just in case they needed it someday". If this is you, do yourself a favor and get rid of these things.

- Bags of bags with extra bags in them. Sure, yes, save a few bags. Like five or ten. Not like 100 or 50 or 30. I mean gift bags, plastic bags, paper bags, cheap cloth bags that you got free from the bank, lunch bags, and any other bag you can think of. Do not hold up a bag and say that you could use it someday just because it is a bag. You won't. You'll use the bag that you like, the one that you always use. This one (and its 100 friends) is taking up your precious space and eating your energy. Get rid of them.
- Potential craft items, because maybe you'll need them. In this instance, I mean complete junk that really would otherwise be labeled as trash. Plastic margarine containers, egg cartons, random buttons, a bag of colorful feathers, googly eyes in

excess, toilet paper rolls, paper towel rolls, cardboard boxes, shoe boxes – you get the idea. Do you have a stash of this stuff somewhere? When did you last use it? If you can't come up with a recent date, it's time to get rid of it. If you no longer have small children at home, keeping these things is a delusional hope that your grandchildren will come over one day and decide to make a craft of a paper towel roll with googly eyes and glitter. Just get rid of it. Really.

- Potentially useful things that were on sale so you bought 100 of them. Are you an eBay store? If so, I guess you can get a pass. If not, please do not clutter up your life and your storage with things like this. It will cost you your space, your energy, and your visual freedom. The chances of you using them are often nil. Be realistic. Saving money is a noble thing, but doing so in a responsible way is better.

- Lids to something you lost nine months ago. If they don't have a partner, why are you keeping them? Same idea for random containers, especially if they're plastic ex-food containers.

- Gifts from someone that you would feel bad about throwing away, but you don't want it and won't use it. I mean, what if they come over and demand to see the ugly sweater that they bought you? What is this, a power-tripping gift hostage situation? If you gave someone a gift and they hated it, would you be pleased with yourself to think that they were keeping it around just so that you weren't offended? I certainly hope not. Do not be held hostage by things or by the thought that people will be offended if you threw it out. It is a gift. Once it belongs to you, you can choose its fate. That's how it works. (Now, if there is some family heirloom of historical value, perhaps you should pawn it off on your sister or someone who would appreciate it more than you, but otherwise, get it gone.) Be thankful that someone thought of you, but do not allow an object to own you.

I am a huge fan of Marie Kondo and the "KonMari" method. Her purging question is simple and cuts to the point. Hold up an object and ask yourself, "Does this spark joy for me?" If it doesn't, throw it away. Everything that you own should be functional and pleasing to you. This is especially useful for clothing. Just because something fits does not mean that you have to keep it. You should be keeping things that you love. It may be that you have to keep one outfit for painting the walls or climbing in mud puddles and hopping fences, but otherwise, imagine what it would feel like to live a life in a simplified manner, surrounded by things that bring you joy and are beautiful to you. It is a freeing thing. It is a wonderful thing to open your closet and to be able to pick anything off of a hanger that you would love to wear today.

Imagine being surrounded in your space by only things that are lovely to you and that bring you joy. Think of the simplicity, the clean feel, the lightness that you could feel in that space. Everything we own has a potential to give to us, but everything we own takes something from us. We must move it, clean it, take care of it, and give it some of our energy. If it isn't bringing you joy, it is taking from you more than it is giving. That doesn't make for a good cost-benefit ratio and is neither logical nor serving you well.

I have spoken with many people who have purged and drastically reduced their belongings, allowing themselves to be surrounded only by things that work for them and that they find beautiful. Their response to this exercise and practice expands and has ripple effects in other areas of their lives – they are more productive (as you can imagine – they don't have to spend a lot of time looking for lost things or shoving things aside to get to other things), they are happier (because their surroundings are clean and beautiful and no longer look like a to-do list), and interestingly enough, I've heard them express that they feel emotionally "lighter".

If you have ever escaped a bad relationship or a bad work environment or resolved a large problem, you can relate to this feeling of emotional release and lightness. It is exciting and encouraging that you may have been bogged down by your things and not even know it – a source of stress that you haven't uncovered. Perhaps you have some stress in your life that is ready to be released through this channel.

One last thing about purging: please be mindful about how many duplicates of things you have. If you really absolutely need four pizza cutters, by all means, keep them, but if you could be honest with yourself and take one step toward a simpler life, you may love the freedom and the benefit of doing so more than the feeling of having three wine bottle openers (even though they look cool). You can't take them with you into eternity (sorry Amenhotep). Keep it all in perspective.

5. Tackle things (as much as possible) as they come instead of procrastinating them.

If you leave all of the little things around the house to do at the end of the day, you've just created a very long (annoying) list of things to do. The small things have just become a big project. Some people really benefit from figuring out how long a task actually takes them to give the motivation to accomplish it right now. If washing the dishes really only takes 3 minutes, you could do that while you're waiting on hold on the phone. If you imagine it to take 20 minutes, you're less likely to want to start it. There is a huge benefit of knowing how long something will take and planning accordingly. Can you vacuum and dust before you have to leave? Could you wash the utensils you chopped the veggies with while the pasta is boiling? As much as you can, tackle those things head on and have a realistic perspective on how long each task takes you.

Now, if you are an organized person, I must ask you to think of something my Aunt Kathy told me – if organizing has begun to interfere with productivity, the goal is lost. You want your space to work for you, not against you. You should own your things, and not the other way around.

Action steps

As you think about spaces and places in your life that you'd like to fine-tune for increased productivity, understand that the physical takes a toll on our emotional and mental health. If you're bogged down, you may need to physically purge. Give yourself the freedom to let go of things. Keep close the things that nurture you and that you love. Time yourself for how long it takes to accomplish tasks. Write it down in a notebook (or on your phone). When you have a few minutes to spare, look at the list and choose productivity. Tackle tasks with vigor and determination, and as they come. Give things a place to live in your home, and when something new comes in, get rid of something old. When you are a consumer, balance yourself and also be a giver. Do not let your stuff own you. Find your balance and rock it. You're the boss of the stuff. Make it work for you.

Chapter 11:
Your Kick in the Rear

Lifetime goal: Improve, change, experiment, tweak, grow. Summon sisu and make stuff happen.

Life has a lot of seasons and ups and downs. As I go through six-month programs with my clients, I get to see the highs and lows and I am honored to walk through the challenges with them and watch them grow. When you are faced with difficulties and you are taking care of yourself, you set yourself up to get the support you need. It is a lot easier to face the giants and the monsters when your brain is functioning optimally and your body is able to exert itself through stressful and difficult situations.

The fact is that rough times will come. Things will happen to you that you wish could be different. You may find yourself in a place that your younger self swore you would never land in, or in a health challenge that you could have never predicted, or in predicaments that you can't quite believe are real. Life is a wild ride and there will be times that you need to just tell yourself to hang on and make it through the next week, the next day, the next twelve hours, or the next thirty minutes and put one foot in front of the other. Some days you will focus on survival and all the lofty goals you had will seem laughable and distant.

I encourage you to hang on. I encourage you in those times to especially to take care of yourself. Do not self-sabotage and dive off of the cliff. It's only harder to be happier the deeper you let yourself go. If you're reading this and you're in one of those times, I understand that it may even be difficult to care. I've been there. I get it. But now is the time - more now than when things are easy – that you need to fight for this.

Get the sleep you need. Drink the water, hydrate your brain. Flush out the toxins. Nourish your body with real food. Take your (whole food based) vitamins and your probiotics. Practice self-care. Be kind to yourself. Talk to yourself instead of listen to yourself. Go get a cup of tea with a friend. Laugh. Disconnect from the madness of social media. Volunteer and pour out your talents for others. Help someone who needs it. Pray. Take a walk outside and look up at the big sky and be thankful for the beautiful things around you that you take for granted. Exercise hard. Love others without regret and freely. When you see something wonderful in someone, say it.

You are unique and you are needed. You have a place in this world and you have talents to give. Imagine if we all lived up to our potential, if we gave it all, and how amazingly different things would look here. I want you to be able to fulfill your calling and your passion. I want you to thrive.

There is a word in Finnish called "*sisu*". It is known to be a central part of what it means to be Finnish and is highly valued for Finns. There is no adequate English equivalent but it may be summed up with a few words: tenacity, grit, perseverance, courage, strength of will, hardiness, endurance, bravery, resilience in the face of insurmountable odds, and pushing past the physical and emotional limits of what you thought you possessed.

In the late fall and early winter of 1939, the Soviet Union invaded Finland in a war that would become known as the Winter War. Stalin and the Red

Army had their eyes on conquest, and little Finland seemed an easy target, a land ready to be mopped up and braided into their empire. Soviet General Meretskov calculated that his army would subdue and take over Finland in ten to twelve days. Just the city of Leningrad alone was the equivalent of the entire Finnish population. The Finnish army was about one-fourth the size of that of the Soviets; they were outnumbered 114 to 3880 in aircraft, and 32 to 6500 in tanks. Finnish soldiers had no uniforms and simply wore their winter clothing, had no anti-aircraft guns or heavy artillery, and although they claimed 32 tanks, only one was properly working.

When the sea of seemingly endless Soviets came into view to destroy the Finns and take over their land, the small haphazard army looked toward their enemy with steely eyes and determination and with dark humor wondered aloud, "There are so many of them and our country is so small, where shall we find room to bury them all?"

With this, the Finns relied on sheer willpower, guerrilla warfare, and mental cunning to defend their country and their lives. They burned everything from bridges, roads, houses, and farms to the ground to prevent the Soviets from having easy access or supplies. The burning was complete, everything reduced to a waste of useless ashes, and among those ashes the Finns planted mines. As they did not have the resources that the Soviets did, they created the Molotov cocktail, an explosive incendiary of petroleum or alcohol, thickened with soap or tar encased in a glass bottle, sometimes wrapped in barbed wire. It was corked and wrapped in a rag that would be dipped and ignited and then thrown so that it would shatter, spill its flammable contents and burn whatever it touched. The Soviet tanks had gasoline engines, and the Molotov cocktails were delivered to these tanks via Finnish daredevils on skis.

One Finnish man, Corporal Simo Häyhä, dressed to be camouflaged in white against the snow and went out as a sniper and took out over 800 Soviets with a bolt-action rifle with open sights routinely at distances of over 400 meters (in the four hours of daylight of the Finnish winter). The Soviets nicknamed him "White Death" and had specific missions that targeted him. One week before the armistice was signed, a Soviet sniper successfully shot him in the face. The bullet crushed his left jaw and blew off his left cheek. Fellow soldiers who evacuated him remarked that "half of his head was missing". He managed to pick up his rifle and finish off the sniper who hit him. Häyhä regained consciousness the day the armistice was signed, and although it took years to recuperate, he did – and lived to be 96 years old.

After 105 exhausting days, the armistice was signed. The Soviets tucked and turned their embarrassed army and went home. A strip of land was annexed to the Soviet Union and twelve percent of Finland's population who lived in that section were given the choice of becoming Soviet subjects or to evacuate to the small strip of land that was left to them. Nearly every single one of them packed up and left their homes, refusing to become subject to Soviet rule. A Soviet general remarked, "We've won just enough ground to bury our dead." (Which is especially fitting and ironic when you think of the initial comments by the Finnish to the Soviet giant that came to attack them at the beginning of the war.)

Finland withstood a giant 51 times its geographic size and made it turn around and flee with one tank, men on skis, Molotov cocktails, the world's best sniper, and the sheer determination to push past and to never give up – not even in the face of what others would deem impossible.

Why on earth am I telling you about the history of Finland? Because, dear one, if such a small one can face a giant and succeed, so can you. What is your giant? Summon your inner sisu and attack with tenacity. This is your life and you can do anything you want to do with it. You have a calling and you have a purpose. Wake yourself up and do it, and do it well and with all of your heart.

There will be many times on your journey that you will self-sabotage or want to give up. You will feel like things aren't working. You will start listening to the voice in your head that tells you that you can't do it. This is normal. Expect it. When those times come, do not let them swallow you up. Get up the next morning and start over. You'll have to step up your game of speaking kindly to yourself and planning ahead, reminding yourself of your goals and why you're doing what you're doing. You are not a quitter. You either win or you learn.

Every little step you take toward your purpose is the right direction. You won't always move in long jumps and gracious leaps, but you've got to walk in the right direction every day.

The sum total of a life changed is marked by just one thing at a time.

Now go, be awesome. I can't wait to see you shine.

thank you

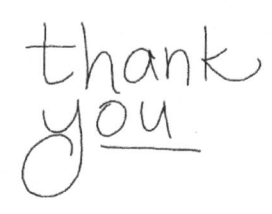

A book a hecking ton of work and it takes a lot of people to help the pieces fit together. I would be remiss not to thank the people who had my back throughout this whole process.

First – Joshua Rosenthal and the staff of the book course (especially the amazing sugar-free Sue Brown, sunshiny Liz Palmieri, and talented Marissa Leigh. P.S. Go buy their books.). Thank you for dreaming big and for making IIN a reality. It was a hand in reaching me to my dreams of becoming an integrative nutrition health coach with a holistic outlook. The whole book course staff are nothing short of driven, passionate, cheerleaders with tons of experience, information, encouragement, and a hand to help all the time. Not only this, but you are quality, fun, and thoughtful people.

Next up, my clients. I spring out of bed every morning excited that I get to work with you and help you iron out issues and celebrate your successes. You're interesting, you make me think, and I am humbled that you trust me and share so much of yourself with me. I do not take it lightly and I carry parts of you in my heart and mind all the time.

I want to thank those people that gave their time to me, reading over my manuscript for errors, for content, and for technical correction – especially my accountability partner, Trecy Marr. The feedback and input that I got from each of you was instrumental in putting out my final version and your comments inspired me, fired me up, and made me hungry (even more than second breakfast) to make this all that I could. You were my team and you had my back on this. Thank you for giving that to me and for making me light up with your encouraging, *amusing*, and helpful comments.

Special thanks to David, Chris, and Michael for helping me with page numbers. It really shouldn't have been that difficult, but yes, I needed three people to get it right. Thank you for being the barricade that prevented me from sliding onto the floor into a frustrated puddle of tears.

The cute chica, Natalie Hindt - thank you for doing my hair and makeup. You are talented and sweet. I love that you knew what I wanted before I said it.

A secret handshake and warm hug to my phenomenal stylists, your eyes and fashion sense bespeak of guru levels. When things take off, I'll hire you daily and send you to Fiji for your bonuses.

A double high five to Chris Amos at Chris Amos Photography, who tolerated my quirky requests, entourages, and Justin Timberlake music while you were working. Your work is incredible. Thank you for making me look way better than I actually do.

Sheeja, I owe many things to you, girlfriend. From fixing my orange (and green) hair, my lumpy shirts, and my eyelashes, to cranking out Lecrae and dance music, to supplying me with tea and love, and for telling me that I needed help and being part of giving that help – you are my sista from anotha mista and my tribe. I love you.

Tess, my dahling, thank you for listening to me and loving me. You have always been my supporter and cheerleader. Tack, bästis. Puss. Jag älskar dej så mycket.

A gigantic hug and thanks to the best graphic designer, Amie Olson. Thank you for being there and bouncing ideas back and forth and for holding my hand through the publishing process. Thank you for pushing me to go where I didn't want to in order to stretch me and make things better and more creative.

A special thank you goes out to my Mom for being the only one who leapt at the chance to red pen me, who incidentally also taught me to love books and reading from a very young age. I knew you would not back down from the opportunity to set things in their proper way, it's the epitome of your life. Obvs. And let's not forget - you're the best seamstress and waffle maker this side of the equator.

Dad, thank you for instilling sisu in me. You're the most capable and uncomplaining person I've ever met. You would win in a fight against Chuck Norris and Rambo – and even at 70, you're a better slalom water-skier than they are (*and* you do it from a jump start with a fancy rooster tail that would make them cry), you make boats by hand, and drag quartered elks up and down mountains for miles like it's no problem.

My dear Kel, thank you for hooking me up with people. You got every single one of the sweet genes (and all the feelings). Thank you for always being an encouragement to me. You're *lit-tra-ly* the best.

Bunny Hop, I figured since I mentioned everyone else that I have to put you in here, but I don't know what for. Just kidding, you're fine. Thanks for your support, which is generally in the form of comedic movie quotes. Do a 360.

Hubster, thank you for encouraging me and telling me that my book was going to be great even before you read it and for always being the nicer and more normal one of the two of us. You're very patient. Like a lot patient. Like the patient-ist. Thanks. Also, you've got great bow and arrow skills, you don't even use sights, and you make delicious grass-fed burgers.

My Football Player, thank you for saying that you're proud of me for writing a book. I love that. You're such a good helper and I can always count on you to clean things up and be responsible – and to let me put my freezing hands on you. That's good stuff, kid.

Thank you to my sweet little Squeaky for being so self-sufficient and self-motivated to do what you had to do so that I could do what I had to do. You're my all-time best blanket getter and you always take such good care of me. I love learning about black holes and science with you.

You peeps are all 100% bomb dot com awesomesauce. I'm thankful that you're all in my life.

And to all of you who read this book, thank you. Really. Thanks for listening to what I had bottled up and wanted to say.

May you get healthy and be happy!

Peace, love, and hugs to all of you,

Keri

Endnotes

[1] Institute of Medicine. Dietary reference intakes for water, potassium, sodium, chloride and sulfate.
http://www.nal.usda.gov/fnic/DRI//DRI_Water/73-185.pdf Accessed 12/12/16

[2] Mullenix, Phyllis J, et al. Neurotoxicity of sodium fluoride in rats.
http://www.sciencedirect.com/science/article/pii/089203629400070T Accessed 2/6/17

[3] Tomljenovic, L. Aluminum and Alzheimer's disease: After a century of controversy, is there a plausible link?
https://www.ncbi.nlm.nih.gov/pubmed/21157018 Accessed 11/22/2016

[4] Holmberg S, Thelin A. High dairy fat intake related to less central obesity: a male cohort study with 12 years' follow-up.
https://www.ncbi.nlm.nih.gov/pubmed/23320900 Accessed 12/26/16

[5] Larson, S C; Wolk, A. Red and Processed Meat Consumption and risk of pancreatic cancer: meta-analysis of prospective studies.
https://www.ncbi.nlm.nih.gov/pmc/articles/PMC3273353/ Accessed 12/28/16

[6] Kilfoy, B A et al. Risk of non-Hodgkin lymphoma and nitrate and nitrite from the diet in Connecticut women.
https://www.ncbi.nlm.nih.gov/pubmed/20204494 Accessed 12/15/16

[7] London, Leslie et al. Neurobehavioral and neurodevelopmental effects of pesticide exposures.
https://www.ncbi.nlm.nih.gov/pmc/articles/PMC3371394/ Accessed 12/29/16

[8] O'Keefe JH, Bhatti SK, Bajwa A, DiNicolantonio JJ, Lavie CJ. Alcohol and cardiovascular health: the dose makes the poison…or the remedy. Mayo Clin Proc. 2014 Mar; 89(3):382-93.

[9] Boffetta, P; Hashibe, M. Cancer and alcohol. https://www.ncbi.nlm.nih.gov/pubmed/16455479 Accessed 1/3/17

[10] Arif AA, Rohrer JE Patterns of alcohol drinking and its association with obesity: data from the Third National Health and Nutrition Examination Survey, 1988-1994. BMC Public Health. 2005 Dec 5; 5():126

[11] Wannamethee SG, Shaper AG, Whincup PH Int J Obes (Lond). Alcohol and adiposity: effects of quantity and type of drink and time relation with meals. 2005 Dec; 29(12):1436-44.

[12] Crocq, Marc-Antoine Alcohol, nicotine, caffeine, and mental disorders. https://www.ncbi.nlm.nih.gov/pmc/articles/PMC3181622/ Accessed 1/3/17

[13] Yu-Jie Zhang, Sha Li, Ren-You Gan, Tong Zhou, Dong-Ping Xu, and Hua-Bin Li. Impacts of Gut Bacteria on Human Health and Diseases. https://www.ncbi.nlm.nih.gov/pmc/articles/PMC4425030,. Accessed 12/12/16

[14] G B Rogers, D J Keating, R L Young, M-L Wong, J Licinio and S Wesselingh. From gut dysbiosis to altered brain function and mental illness: mechanisms and pathways. www.nature.com/mp/journal/v21/n6/full/mp201650a.html Accessed 12/13/16

[15] Miyoshi M, Ogawa A, Higurashi S, Kadooka Y. Anti-obesity effect of Lactobacillus gasseri SBT2055 accompanied by inhibition of pro-inflammatory gene expression in the visceral adipose tissue in diet-induced obese mice. https://www.ncbi.nlm.nih.gov/pubmed/23917447 Accessed 12/15/16

[16] Ahlskog, Eric J. et al. Physical Exercise as a Preventive or Disease-Modifying Treatment of Dementia and Brain Aging https://www.ncbi.nlm.nih.gov/pmc/articles/PMC3258000/ Accessed 12/20/16

[17] Ahlskog, Eric J. et al. Physical Exercise as a Preventative or Disease-Modifying Treatment of Dementia and Brain Aging https://www.ncbi.nlm.nih.gov/pmc/articles/PMC3258000/ Accessed 12/21/16

[18] Ashish Sharma, M.D., Vishal Madaan, M.D., and Frederick D. Petty, M.D., Ph.D. Exercise for Mental Health https://www.ncbi.nlm.nih.gov/pmc/articles/PMC1470658/, Accessed 12/19/16

[19] . McNeil JK, LeBlanc EM, Joyner M. The effect of exercise on depressive symptoms in the moderately depressed elderly Psychol Aging. 1991 Sep; 6(3):487-8.

[20] Hannah Steinberg, Moss, Sykes, Lowery, Dewey, LeBoutillier. Short exercise enhances creativity independently of mood. http://bjsm.bmj.com/content/31/3/240., *Br J Sports Med 1997* Accessed 12/26/16

[21] Peterson, D. Anxious or feeling down: can essential oils help? http://info.achs.edu/blog/depression-and-anxiety-can-essential-oils-help#_ftnref2 Accessed 1/4/2017

[22] Chang, S.Y. (2008). Effects of aroma hand massage on pain, state anxiety and depression in hospice patients with terminal cancer. *Taehan Kanho Hakhoe Chi.*, 38(4):493-502.

[23] Chang, K. & Shen, C. (2011). Aromatherapy Benefits Autonomic Nervous System Regulation for Elementary School Faculty in Taiwan. *Evidence-Based Complementary and Alternative Medicine*

[24] Shiina Y., Funabashi N., Lee K., Toyoda T., Sekine T., Honjo S., et al. (2007). Relaxation effects of lavender aromatherapy improve coronary flow velocity reserve in healthy men evaluated by transthoracic Doppler echocardiography. *Int J Cardiol.*, 129(2):193-7.

[25] Woelk, H. & Schläfke, S. (2010). A multi-center, double- blind, randomized study of the Lavender oil preparation Silexan in comparison to Lorazepam for generalized anxiety disorder. *Phytomedicine,* 17(2):94-9.

[26] Dew et al, 2008. Religion/Spirituality and adolescent psychiatric symptoms: a review. http://www.ncbi.nlm.nih.gov/pubmed/18219572. Accessed 1/5/17

[27] T. Field, , M. Hemandez-Reif, S. Taylor, O. Quintino & I. Burman. Labor pain is reduced by massage therapy.

http://www.tandfonline.com/doi/abs/10.3109/01674829709080701 Accessed 1/5/17.

[28] Steptoe, Andrew et al. Black tea soothes away stress. https://www.ucl.ac.uk/media/library/tea Accessed 1/5/17

[29] Shift Work and Cancer. https://www.ncbi.nlm.nih.gov/pmc/articles/PMC2954516/ Thomas C Erren, Prof. Dr. med., Puran Falaturi, Prof. Dr. med., Peter Morfeld, PD Dr. rer. medic., Peter Knauth, Prof. Dr.-Ing., Russel J Reiter, Prof. Dr. rer. nat. Dr. h. c. mult., and Claus Piekarski, Prof. em. Dr. med

[30] Breslau, N. et al., Sleep Disturbance and Psychiatric Disorders: A Longitudinal Epidemiological Study of Young Adults, Biological Psychiatry. Mar 1996; 39(6): 411–418.

[31] https://www.ncbi.nlm.nih.gov/pmc/articles/PMC535701/ Short Sleep Duration is Associated with Reduced Leptin, Elevated Ghrelin, and Increased Body Mass Index, Shahrad Taheri,, et al., accessed 1/19/17

[32] https://www.ncbi.nlm.nih.gov/pubmed/9415946 Sleep loss results in an elevation of cortisol levels the next evening. Leproult R. et al., accessed 1/19/17

[33] https://www.ncbi.nlm.nih.gov/pubmed/24435056 The relationship between sleep disorders and testosterone in men. Wittert G., accessed 1/19/17

[34] Thakkar, M. et al. Alcohol disrupts sleep homeostasis. https://www.ncbi.nlm.nih.gov/pmc/articles/PMC4427543/ Accessed 1/20/17

[35] http://science.sciencemag.org/content/221/4606/182 Physiological correlates of prolonged sleep deprivation in rats. Rechtschaffen, A. et al. Accessed 1/20/17

[36] Strean, William. Laughter Prescription. https://www.ncbi.nlm.nih.gov/pmc/articles/PMC2762283/ Accessed 1/23/17

[37] Hayashi, K. et al. Laughter Lowered the Increase of Postprandial Blood Glucose http://care.diabetesjournals.org/content/26/5/1651 Accessed 1/23/17

This page intentionally left blank for you to write math problems on.

Made in the USA
Monee, IL
08 December 2019